U0287152

山东大学精品立项教材 供口腔医学类专业使用

牙体缺损修复
备牙过程图解

Atlas of the Preparation Process for Tooth Defect Restoration

主 编 蓝 菁 林 东 葛少华

科学出版社

北 京

内 容 简 介

本书在整合口腔修复专业教材的基础上，详尽介绍了前/后牙全瓷冠、贴面、嵌体等临床常用修复体的牙体预备过程，以图文＋视频形式展示整个预备步骤、操作要求和技巧，直观展示整个过程。同时提供英文对照，有助于口腔医学生及青年医师学习专业英语。

本书图片清晰、操作规范、步骤详细，可供口腔医学生、住培医师参考。

图书在版编目（CIP）数据

牙体缺损修复备牙过程图解／蓝菁，林东，葛少华主编．—北京：科学出版社，2021.6

ISBN 978-7-03-067301-5

Ⅰ．①牙…　Ⅱ．①蓝…②林…③葛…　Ⅲ．①牙体 – 修复术 – 图解　Ⅳ．① R781.05-64

中国版本图书馆 CIP 数据核字（2020）第 253551 号

责任编辑：马晓伟／责任校对：杨　赛
责任印制：霍　兵／封面设计：龙　岩

科 学 出 版 社 出版

北京东黄城根北街16号
邮政编码：100717
http://www.sciencep.com

北京汇瑞嘉合文化发展有限公司印刷
科学出版社发行　各地新华书店经销

*

2021年 6 月第 一 版　开本：787×1092　1/16
2023年 4 月第四次印刷　印张：9
字数：193 000

定价：88.00元

（如有印装质量问题，我社负责调换）

主 编 简 介

蓝菁 主任医师，博士生导师，美国加州大学旧金山分校牙学院博士后，山东大学口腔医学院修复教研所所长。擅长牙体缺损、牙列缺损、牙列缺失等疾病的诊断治疗及疑难病例的多学科联合治疗；致力于功能与美学的修复治疗。主要从事高脂血症与骨结合的相关性研究、种植体材料改性及种植体周围炎疫苗的研究。主持国家自然科学基金项目2项，省级课题4项，山东大学交叉学科项目2项。以第一或通讯作者发表SCI论文17篇。获批国家发明专利2项。获2018年度山东省科技进步奖二等奖（第二位）。担任国家自然科学基金同行评议专家、《口腔医学》审稿专家。

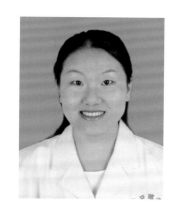

林东 山东大学口腔医院副主任医师，中华口腔医学会口腔美学专委会青年委员、工作秘书及青年讲师，中华口腔医学会种植专委会会员，山东省口腔美学专委会委员兼学会秘书，中华口腔医学会"一步一步"项目讲师，北京大学口腔医院进修美学修复获"北京大学优秀学员"，齿美教育青年讲师。主持厅级教研项目1项，主编国家级本科实验教材1部，连续四年进入全国美学病例大赛决赛及在全国"一步一步"操作大赛中获奖。

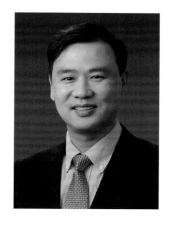

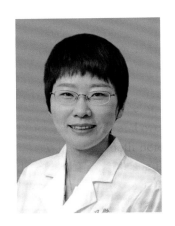

葛少华 教授，博士生导师，山东大学口腔医院主任医师，泰山学者特聘专家，中华口腔医学会牙周专委会常委，教育部高等学校口腔医学专业教学指导委员会委员，中国卫生信息与健康医疗大数据学会口腔医学专业委员会副主任委员，中华口腔医学会口腔科研管理分会常委，中华口腔医学会口腔医学教育专委会常委，全国宝钢基金优秀教师，山东省十佳女医师，山东省中青年优秀保健人才。担任《口腔医学》副主编，*ACS AMI*、*J Dent Res* 等审稿人，国家自然科学基金同行评议专家，省部级科学技术奖评审专家。主要研究方向为牙周组织发育与再生，主持国家自然科学基金项目4项、省部级课题5项。获山东省优秀教学成果奖二等奖1项，山东省科技进步奖二等奖1项，山东省医学科技奖二等奖2项，山东省高等学校优秀科研成果奖三等奖1项。在国内外专业期刊上发表论文100余篇，其中以第一或通讯作者发表SCI论文38篇；主编著作1部。

《牙体缺损修复备牙过程图解》
编写人员

主　　编　蓝　菁　林　东　葛少华

副 主 编　孙钦峰　孙圣军　马　丽　高　旭

编　　者　（按姓氏笔画排序）

马　丽　　冯丹丹　　刘奇博　　祁　冬

孙圣军　　孙钦峰　　李传花　　宋　珊

宋理想　　张广灿　　张玉军　　陈井春雨

林　东　　郑　政　　赵　凌　　高　旭

郭美画　　葛少华　　蓝　菁

编写秘书　郭美画

序　一

  牙体缺损的修复是口腔修复中的重要组成部分，其中精准的牙体预备是基础，直接影响后续治疗的质量和修复体的使用寿命，是每个口腔医师必须掌握的基本功之一。牙体预备是实践性非常强的环节，虽然众多口腔修复学教材中均有介绍，但多以文字描述为主。牙体预备应选用什么器械、怎么磨、磨多少，初学者和年轻医师往往对此感到非常迷茫。

  很欣慰我的母校山东大学口腔医学院有一批优秀、敬业的同行，他们合作编写了《牙体缺损修复备牙过程图解》一书。该书以图文形式呈现牙体预备的操作步骤、操作要求、操作技巧，并配合视频，使整个过程跃然纸上，以便于初学者与年轻医师理解和掌握。书中详尽介绍了临床最常用修复体类型的牙体预备方法，包括前/后牙的全瓷冠、贴面及嵌体等，对于住培医师的培养、年轻医师操作的规范化都有很好的指导作用。同时，该书配有英文对照，可以加强口腔医学生及青年医师专业英语的学习。

  教学是每个口腔医学院的根本，作为高等医学院校的教师，努力培养医学人才是我们的责任和使命。非常高兴看到蓝菁教授、林东教授所带领的山东大学口腔医学院口腔修复教研所，始终能够牢记使命、不忘初心，孜孜不倦、踏踏实实地做好教学工作。他们在口腔修复学的教学内容和教学形式上进行了大力改革，并取得可喜成绩，该书就是他们教学改革的成果之一。"为天下储人才，为国家图富强"是山东大学的办学宗旨，我为母校能够始终以本科教学为根本，为国家培养了大批优秀口腔医学人才感到自豪。最后，特别感谢广大读者朋友们的支持，希望大家通过该书能够收获更多临床实用知识。

徐世同

2020 年 6 月

序 二

　　牙体缺损的修复是口腔各类修复形式的基础，常用牙体缺损的修复形式有全冠、贴面和嵌体，其牙体预备的好坏关系到修复体的质量和长期预后。可以说，牙体预备是修复医师的重要临床基本功之一，也是口腔修复学教学的难点和重点。《牙体缺损修复备牙过程图解》一书通过图文和视频的形式展示了牙体缺损常见修复体的详细操作过程，与教学内容相辅相成，相得益彰，是一本难得的教学和临床辅助用书。

　　该书全面介绍了前/后牙全瓷冠、各类贴面和嵌体的牙体预备过程，内容涵盖了车针的选择、邻面的打开、牙体去除量等精准控制技巧，各个细节均以与图文结合的形式呈现，直观清晰、实用性强。该书内容全面，操作步骤规范、详细、便于本科生、研究生和规培学员理解，对其掌握规范的牙体预备过程有着重要的指导作用。

　　作为一名高年资修复医师和教师，我非常高兴看到该书的出版。山东大学口腔医学院以蓝菁教授为首的修复教研室同仁们对教学工作精益求精的精神、认真负责的态度和扎实的临床技能，值得我们学习。

2020 年 6 月

前　言

　　2020 年初，我们经历了一场全国上下同心协力抗击新型冠状病毒的战役，使我们的心灵再一次受到洗涤，同时也提醒了我们，作为一名医务工作者和教师，只有在日常工作中未雨绸缪，面对突如其来、复杂多变的情况时才会有足够的信心。

　　近几年，随着材料学、机械学、信息学等的不断发展，口腔修复学也快速进步，各种新材料、新设备层出不穷，但牙体预备仍是口腔修复中最基本的操作环节。在多年的教学工作中我们发现，牙体预备一直是困扰学生们的重点和难点之一，也是每个口腔医师职业生涯的起点。以文字介绍为主，靠学生们在有限的实验课时间和以后的执业过程中不断摸索和提高的教学模式，已不能完全适应当代口腔医学生和年轻医师培养的要求。当前，我们急需符合口腔医学生及初学者需求的图文视听教材，以便使他们在一开始就能接受更易理解和掌握的规范化培养。山东大学大力加强本科教学的投入，口腔医学院更是将本科教学提升至战略发展目标，口腔修复教研所借教育改革的东风，不断进行教学改革、提升教学能力，这个过程中《牙体缺损修复备牙过程图解》应运而生。本书集文字、图片及视频于一体，内容涵盖牙体缺损常见修复体类型的牙体预备过程，包括前牙、后牙全瓷冠牙体预备，前牙三种经典瓷贴面牙体预备，以及后牙瓷嵌体、高嵌体牙体预备；通过图文和视频形式将每个步骤的要点，以及高效和规范化的预备方法展现给读者；同时提供英文对照，以满足读者的不同学习需求。全书文字描述细致、图片精美、视频清晰，可极大补充我们的教学内容，提高教学效率，有助于口腔医学生、住培医师规范化操作能力的提高。

　　本书在编写过程中得到了山东大学口腔医学院领导、同事们的大力支持，特此表示感谢。由于我们能力有限，书中可能存在疏漏，在此恳请读者们批评指正，以便再版时改进。

主　编

2020 年 12 月

致　谢

　　得益于诸位编者及其家人和朋友的大力支持，本书才得以顺利完成和出版。在这里，我们真诚地感谢你们，是你们的无私奉献和付出，我们才能专心致志地完成如此有意义的工作。

　　首先，特别感谢各位编者的家人。在 2020 年疫情期间，你们给予了莫大的耐心和支持，使我们有足够的时间反复斟酌和完善书中内容，从而使其完美地呈现出来。

　　其次，特别感谢我们的同事和朋友。感谢山东大学口腔医学院的吕波书记对本书给予的重要支持和肯定，使我们有更大的前进动力；感谢教学实验室的李振玉老师、张凯丽老师、吴笑至老师对书中操作及视频录制提供的场所和帮助；感谢教学办公室的芮艳华老师、曹琳老师对本书版式提供的帮助；感谢修复教研所的全体同仁在本书编写过程中给予的大力支持和帮助。

　　特别感谢山东大学及口腔医学院对于本科教学工作的重视，提供诸多教改项目（2019Y260、2019Y264、2019Y257、qlyxjy-202029、2020Y140、2020Y141），为我们提供发展机会和经费支持，使我们在日常教学工作中不断改进、提升。

　　特别感谢卡瓦集团 KaVa Kerr 事业部提供的器械和材料，使我们的操作得心应手。

　　再次感谢大家，正是你们的支持和帮助，本书才得以顺利出版。

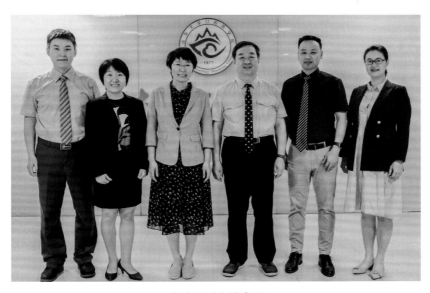

主编及副主编合影

目　录

CONTENTS

第一章　牙体缺损概述

牙体缺损（tooth defect）是口腔科最常见的疾病之一，是指由于各种原因引起的牙体硬组织不同程度的外形、结构及颜色的破坏和异常，表现为牙体失去了正常的解剖学外形和颜色，对牙髓、牙周组织、咀嚼、发音、面容，甚至对全身健康都会产生不同程度的影响。

牙体缺损较小时可以采用直接充填法治疗，但如果剩余牙体组织薄弱，无法为充填体提供良好的固位，剩余牙体组织抗力不足、充填体强度不足或者为了实现更高的美学诉求时，则需要采用修复治疗的方法。牙体缺损的修复是用间接法制作的人工修复体恢复缺损牙的形态、美观和功能，包括嵌体、贴面、部分冠、全冠和桩核冠等。

修复体是一个应用于人体口腔内的机械装置，应满足生物学原则、生物力学原则和美学原则。三原则贯穿于牙体缺损修复治疗的每个阶段，不能过分强调其中的单一方面，否则会影响其他原则的实现，在进行牙体缺损修复的设计时，要综合分析、具体评价。

本书内容就是在综合考虑修复治疗三原则的基础上，设计和实施牙体缺损修复的牙体预备部分。

Chapter 1　Summary of Tooth Defect

The tooth defect is one of the most common manifestation of dental disease. Tooth defect is defined as the destruction and abnormity of the shape, color and tooth structure caused by various reasons. It shows that the tooth has lost its normal anatomical shape and color, which has a different degree of impact on chewing, pronunciation, dental pulp, periodontal tissue, facial appearance and even on the general health.

When the tooth defect is small, it can be treated by direct composite filling. However, if the residual tooth tissue is thin and can not provide enough retention for filling, or the resistance of the residual tissue is lack, or the strength of the filling is not enough, or to achieve a better esthetics appearance, the restoration treatment is needed. The restoration of the tooth defect is to fabricate artificial restoration in indirect process to recover the contour, esthetics and function of the defected tooth, which includes inlay, veneer, partial crown, full-crown and post-core crown.

The dental restoration is a mechanical device applied on human oral, the design of which must be in line with the multifaceted biological, biomechanical and esthetic principles. These three fundamental principles should be applied well through each step from treatment plan design to operation procedure. If we overemphasize one of the three principles, it may interfere in the others. In this way, a comprehensive and concrete analysis is needed when you design the process of restoring the tooth defect.

Based on comprehensive consider of three principles, this book designs and implements the tooth preparation of the defective tooth restoration.

第二章　前牙全瓷冠牙体预备

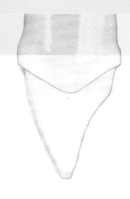

　　全冠是牙体缺损修复治疗中适应范围最广的一种修复体，覆盖整个缺损患牙的所有轴面和𬌗面，可以用来修复缺损患牙的形态、功能和美观；在前牙区，还可用于轻度排列不齐或者扭转牙的美学修复。

　　前牙除具有咀嚼和发音功能外，更重要的功能是美观，因此具备良好美学性能的全瓷冠受到越来越多患者的青睐，临床应用日益广泛。本章就以 21 牙经典的双层结构全瓷冠——氧化锆加饰的全瓷冠牙体预备（预备流程及预备量见图 2-1）为例进行图文视听讲解。

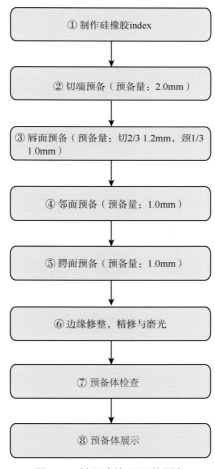

① 制作硅橡胶index

② 切端预备（预备量：2.0mm）

③ 唇面预备（预备量：切2/3 1.2mm，颈1/3 1.0mm）

④ 邻面预备（预备量：1.0mm）

⑤ 腭面预备（预备量：1.0mm）

⑥ 边缘修整，精修与磨光

⑦ 预备体检查

⑧ 预备体展示

图 2-1　前牙全瓷冠牙体预备

Chapter 2　Preparation of All-Ceramic Crown of Anterior Tooth

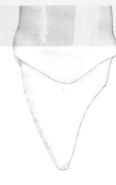

All-ceramic crown is the most popular type of crown used in the dental defects prosthodontic treatment. It covers all the axial and occlusal surfaces of the defected tooth. It can effectively repair the contour, function and aesthetic of the defected tooth. For the anterior, it especially corrects the slight malalinement and torsiversion of the anterior tooth.

The anterior tooth has the function of mastication, pronunciation and more importantly esthetics. Therefore, the all-ceramic crown possessing good esthetic performance is popular increasingly. And it is widely used in clinic growingly. The chapter describes the two layer structure zirconia with decorative porcelain all-ceramic crown which takes the 21 tooth as an example (the procedure and reduction are shown in Fig 2-1) in the form of figure, text and audiovisual instruction.

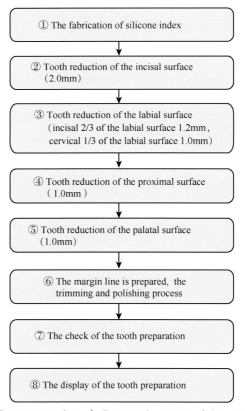

Fig 2-1　The preparation of all-ceramic crown of the anterior tooth

一、制作硅橡胶 index

开始牙体预备前使用加成反应硅橡胶油泥混合型制作 index（图 2-2），唇侧盖过牙龈缘且不影响就位，腭侧制作背板，便于检查腭侧预备量并起固位作用，两侧包绕至预备牙近远中至少两个牙位，index 需制作 2 个，用于显露预备牙不同的位置。

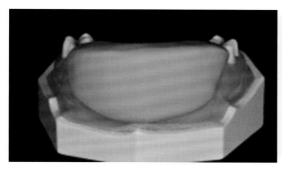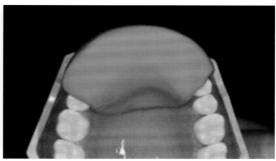

图 2-2 牙体预备前制作 index

严格按照硅橡胶说明书上的硬固时间（一般 4～5min），待硅橡胶硬固后取下，其中一个 index（index-I）用手术刀片沿 21 预备牙正中唇向垂直切开（图 2-3），可以用于检查唇面预备量及预备体形态。

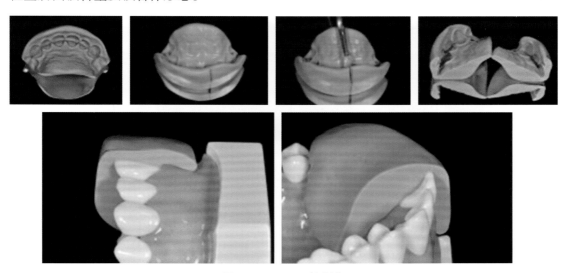

图 2-3 index-I 的制作

1. Fabrication of Silicone Index

Before the tooth preparation, use additional type silicone putty to fabricate two silicone indexes(Fig 2-2). This index extends over the labial gingival edge without interfering with the placement, the palatal side of which is fabricated as the backplane for checking the reduction and providing retention, the proximal side should include at least two other adjacent teeth. Two indexes are made for exposing different parts of the preparation.

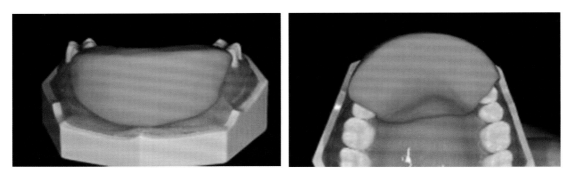

Fig 2-2   Fabricate a silicone index before the tooth preparation

According to the setting time of the instruction(4-5minutes), put out the putty when it gets hard. To check the facial and palatal reduction，one index(index-I) is cut vertically along the midline labiopalatine direction of the 21 tooth(Fig 2-3).

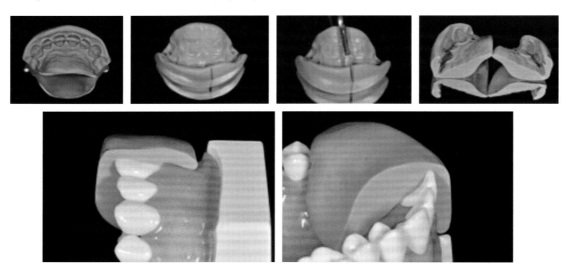

Fig 2-3   The fabrication of index-I

另一个 index（index-Ⅱ）采用开窗式设计（图 2-4），用手术刀片沿图中画线处切开，完全暴露唇侧和切端，用于检查切端预备量。

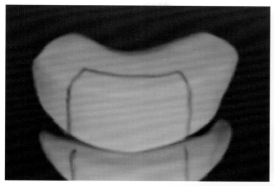
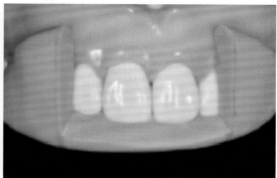
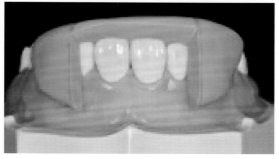

图 2-4　index-Ⅱ的制作

二、切端预备

完成 index 制作后开始进行牙体预备，首先是切端预备。使用直径 1.0mm 的圆头柱状金刚砂车针沿原来切端磨耗斜面的方向切入牙体组织，深度约 2.0mm，相当于车针直径的 2 倍（图 2-5），或者没入两根车针的量。

按照图 2-5 的方法在切端完成 2 ～ 3 条深度指示沟（图 2-6）。

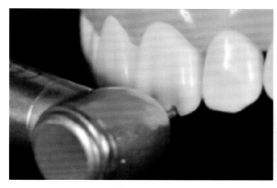
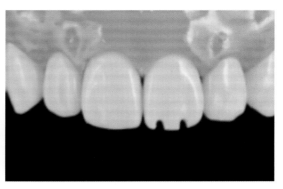

图 2-5　切端 2.0mm 深度指示沟　　　　图 2-6　完成切端指示沟

The other index (index-II) adopts the window type design(Fig 2-4). Use the scalpel to cut along the drawing line to expose the labial surface and incisal edge for checking the incisal edge reduction.

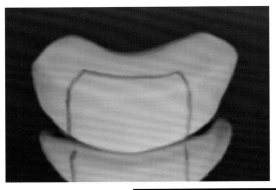
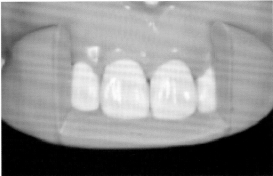

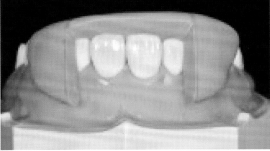

Fig 2-4   The fabrication of index-II

2. Preparation of Incisal Edge

The tooth reduction follows the fabrication of the index. The first step is the preparation of the incisal edge. A 1.0mm diameter round-end cylindrical diamond bur is sunk into tissue along the inclination of the uncut incisal edge to make grooves with the depth of 2.0mm，almost twice of the length of the bur diameter(Fig 2-5)，or to sink two bur depth into the tooth.

2-3 incisal depth orientation grooves are prepared according to the methods of Fig 2-5(Fig 2-6).

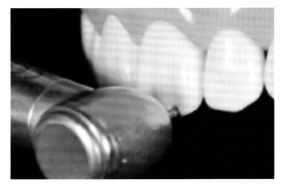
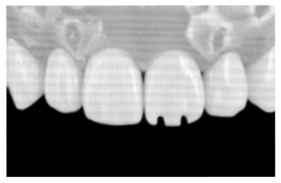

Fig 2-5   2.0mm deep incisal depth grooves   Fig 2-6   Incisal depth grooves are finished

使用探针检查指示沟深度为 2.0mm（图 2-7）。

在完成 2～3 条切端深度指示沟后，使用同一车针沿着原来切端的走行，磨除切端远中切角到远中深度指示沟之间的牙体组织（图 2-8），避免伤及邻牙。

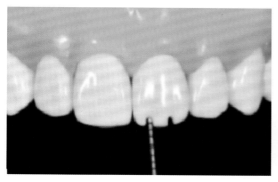 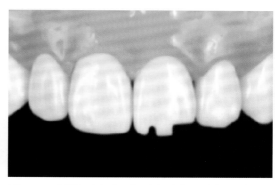

图 2-7　检查指示沟深度　　　　　　图 2-8　磨除远中切角到远中深度指示沟间牙体组织

按照图 2-8 的方法磨除切端其他深度指示沟之间的牙体组织（图 2-9）。预备后的切端，近远中走行与原来的切端平行，唇腭向与原来的磨耗斜面平行（图 2-10）。

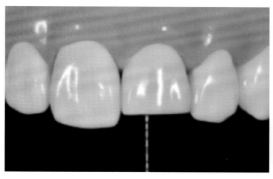 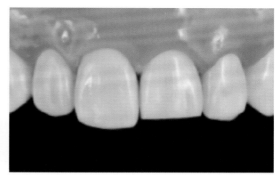

图 2-9　磨除切端其他深度指示沟之间的牙体组织　　　图 2-10　预备后近远中走行与原来的切端平行

切端预备完成后，戴入 index-Ⅱ，确认磨除量为 2.0mm（图 2-11）。

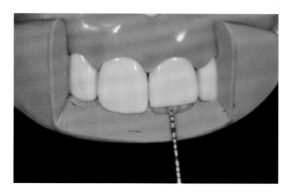

图 2-11　确认切端磨除量

切端预备

Use the periodontal probe to examine the 2.0mm depth of these depth grooves(Fig 2-7).

When the 2-3 depth grooves are finished，the same bur is following the original incisal direction to cut the tissue between distal incisal angle and distal depth groove (Fig 2-8). Take care not to damage the adjacent tooth.

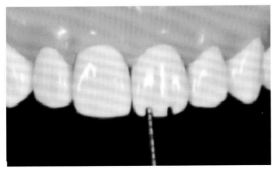

Fig 2-7 Examine the depth of orientation grooves

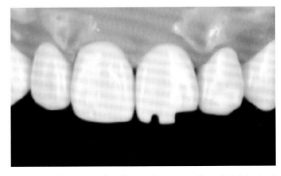

Fig 2-8 Remove the tissue between the distal-incisal angle and distal depth groove

The tissue between other grooves is removed as methods of Fig 2-8(Fig 2-9). The preparation follows the uncut incisal line in mesiodistal direction(Fig 2-10)，which is parallel to the uncut slope in facial-lingual direction.

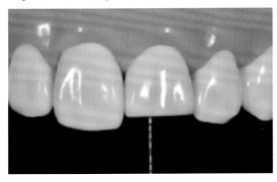

Fig 2-9 Remove the tissue between other grooves

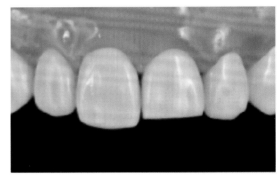

Fig 2-10 Incisal reduction parallels the uncut incisal edge

When the incisal edge preparation is finished, put it into the index-II to make sure the 2.0 reduction (Fig 2-11).

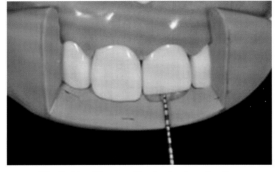

Fig 2-11 Ensure the incisal reduction

三、唇面预备

上中切牙唇面预备须按照切 2/3 与颈 1/3 两个轴面分别预备，以保留上中切牙原有的解剖外形轮廓。首先使用直径 1.0mm 的圆头柱状金刚砂车针，沿与唇面切 2/3 轴面平行的方向切入牙体组织制备深度指示沟，深度为 1.0mm，车针恰好完全没入（图 2-12）。从侧面观，车针放置方向与唇面切 2/3 轴面平行（图 2-13）。

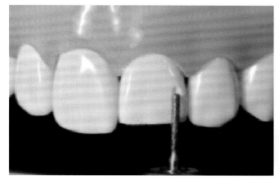

图 2-12　制备唇面切 2/3 指示沟

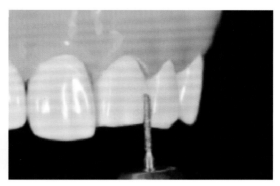

图 2-13　唇面切 2/3 指示沟侧面观

按照图 2-13 的方法，在唇面切 2/3 轴面预备 3 条深度指示沟（图 2-14）。从侧面观，车针方向均与唇面切 2/3 轴面平行切入牙体组织（图 2-15）。

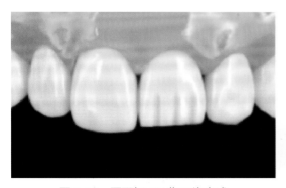

图 2-14　唇面切 2/3 指示沟完成

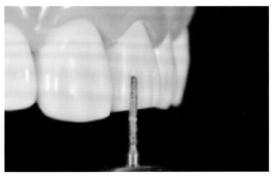

图 2-15　唇面切 2/3 指示沟完成侧面观

3. Preparation of Labial Surface

The tooth reduction of the labial surface is prepared by two parts: the incisal 2/3 axial surface and the cervical 1/3 axial surface separately, which keeps the original anatomical contour of the maxillary incisal tooth. Firstly, a 1.0mm diameter round-end cylindrical diamond is used. The bur is sunk into the tissue, parallel to the incisal 2/3 of the labial surface of the tooth to make the depth grooves. The depth of these grooves is 1.0mm, actually the diamond is inserted into the tooth to its full diameter(Fig 2-12). On the lateral view, the direction of the bur is parallel to the incisal 2/3 of the labial surface(Fig 2-13).

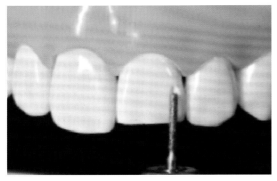

Fig 2-12　Prepare the incisal 2/3 depth grooves on labial surface

Fig 2-13　The lateral view of the depth grooves on the incisal 2/3 of the labial surface

Three depth grooves on the incisal 2/3 of the labial surface are prepared according to the methods of Fig 2-13（Fig 2-14）. On the lateral view, the direction of the bur parallels the incisal 2/3 of the labial surface when the bur cuts into the tooth（Fig 2-15）.

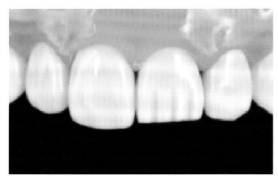
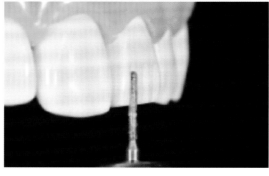

Fig 2-14　The depth grooves on the incisal 2/3 of the labial surface is finished

Fig 2-15　The lateral view of the finished depth grooves on the incisal 2/3 of the labial surface

从切端观（图 2-16）：切 2/3 深度指示沟完全顺应唇面切 2/3 的解剖外形。使用直径 1.0mm 的圆头柱状金刚砂车针，沿与唇面颈 1/3 平行的方向切入牙体组织预备深度指示沟，深度为 1.0mm，车针恰好完全没入（图 2-17）。从侧面观，车针的放置方向与颈 1/3 轴面平行（图 2-18）。

按照图 2-18 的方法，在唇面颈 1/3 轴面预备两条深度指示沟（图 2-19）。

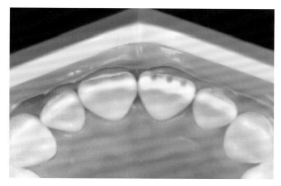

图 2-16　唇面切 2/3 指示沟切端观

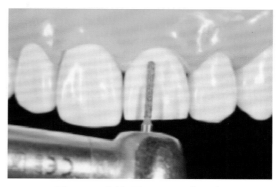

图 2-17　制备唇面颈 1/3 指示沟

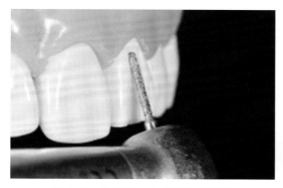

图 2-18　唇面颈 1/3 指示沟侧面观

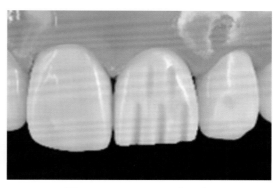

图 2-19　唇面颈 1/3 指示沟

唇面深度指示沟预备完成的切端观（图 2-20）。

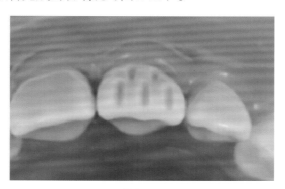

图 2-20　唇面深度指示沟预备完成切端观

On the incisal view(Fig 2-16)，the depth grooves of the incisal 2/3 surface follow the anatomical contour of the tooth completely. A 1.0mm diameter round-end cylindrical diamond is used. The bur is parallel to the cervical 1/3 of the labial surface to cut into the tooth for making the depth grooves. The grooves are 1.0mm deep，exactly the diamond is inserted into the tooth to its full diameter(Fig 2-17). On the lateral view，the direction of the bur is parallel to the cervical 1/3 of the labial surface(Fig 2-18).

Two depth grooves on cervical 1/3 of the labial surface are prepared according to the methods of Fig 2-18(Fig 2-19).

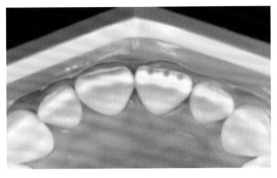

Fig 2-16　The incisal view of the grooves on the incisal 2/3 of the labial surface

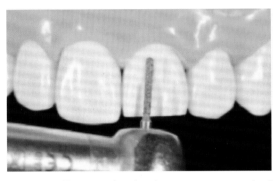

Fig 2-17　Prepare the depth grooves on cervical 1/3

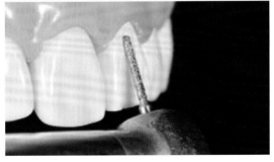

Fig 2-18　The lateral view of the depth grooves on cervical 1/3 of the labial surface

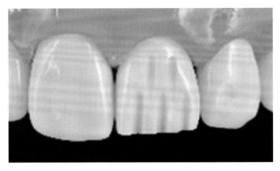

Fig 2-19　The depth grooves on cervical 1/3 of the labial surface

The incisal view of the finished preparation of the labial depth grooves(Fig 2-20).

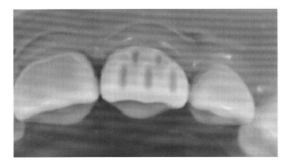

Fig 2-20　The incisal view of the finished depth grooves on labial surface

　　然后更换直径 1.4mm 的圆头柱状金刚砂车针，沿与唇面切 2/3 轴面平行的方向均匀磨除远中边缘嵴至中间深度指示沟之间的牙体组织（图 2-21），磨除边缘嵴时避免伤及邻牙。

　　侧面观，车针放置方向与切 2/3 轴面平行（图 2-22）。

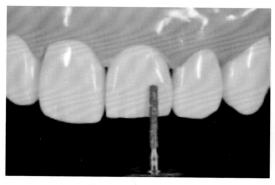

图 2-21　磨除切 2/3 远中边缘嵴至中间深度指示
　　　　　沟之间的牙体组织

图 2-22　侧面观

　　唇面观（图 2-23）。

　　切端观（图 2-24）。

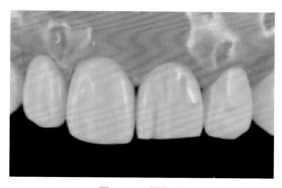
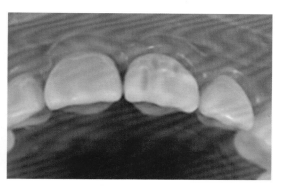

图 2-23　唇面观

图 2-24　切端观

　　按照图 2-21 的方法，沿与唇面切 2/3 轴面平行的方向，均匀磨除中间深度指示沟至近中边缘嵴之间的牙体组织（图 2-25）。切端观（图 2-26）。

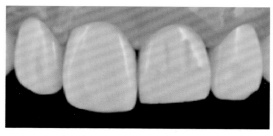
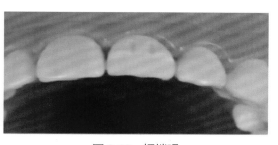

图 2-25　磨除切 2/3 中间深度指示沟至近中边缘
　　　　　嵴之间的牙体组织

图 2-26　切端观

Then，the bur is replaced by a 1.4mm diameter round-end cylindrical diamond，which is parallel to the incisal 2/3 labial surface. Tooth structure between distal marginal ridge to middle depth grooves is removed evenly(Fig 2-21). Take care not to damage the adjacent tooth when preparing the marginal ridge 2/3.

On the lateral view，the direction of the bur is parallel to the incisal 2/3 of the axial surface(Fig 2-22).

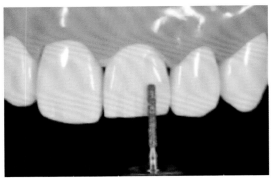

Fig 2-21　Remove the tissue between distal marginal ridge and depth grooves on incisal 2/3 surface

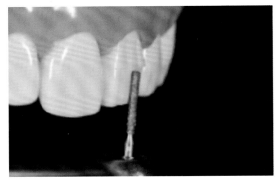

Fig 2-22　The lateral view

The labial view(Fig 2-23).
The incisal view(Fig 2-24).

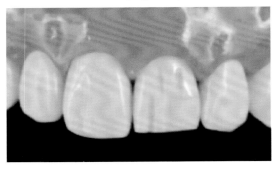

Fig 2-23　The labial view

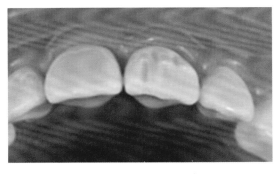

Fig 2-24　The incisal view

As the method of Fig 2-21，the bur is parallel to the incisal 2/3 labial surface. Tooth structure between the middle depth groove and mesial marginal ridge is removed evenly(Fig 2-25). The incisal view(Fig 2-26).

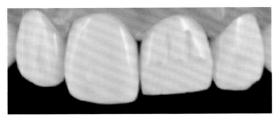

Fig 2-25　Remove the tissue between mesial marginal ridge and the middle depth grooves

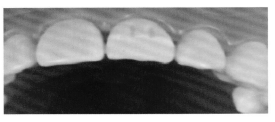

Fig 2-26　The incisal view

　　按照预备唇面切 2/3 的预备方法，使用同一车针沿与唇面颈 1/3 轴面平行的方向，以深度指示沟为参考，磨除颈 1/3 远中到近中的牙体组织，预备时避免伤及邻牙。此时在颈部预备出唇面的颈部边缘线，边缘线位置在平齐龈缘处，宽度为 1.0mm，形态为内线角圆钝的浅凹形边缘线，走行完全顺应牙龈缘的扇贝形外观（图 2-27）。

　　侧面观，车针放置方向与颈 1/3 轴面平行（图 2-28）。

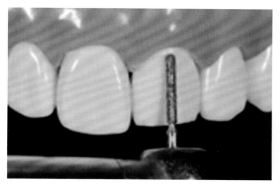
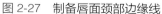

图 2-27　制备唇面颈部边缘线

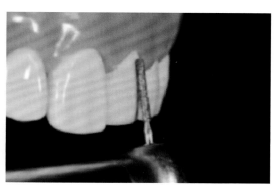

图 2-28　侧面观

　　唇面预备完成，完成的唇侧预备体形态与原牙的解剖轮廓一致（图 2-29），切 2/3 与颈 1/3 的两个预备面平滑相交。在近远中边缘嵴处牙体预备尽量向邻接区扩展，但避免伤及邻牙。

　　唇面预备完成切端观（图 2-30）。

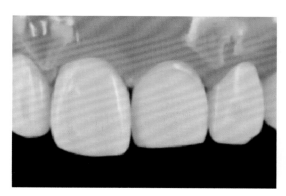

图 2-29　唇面预备完成

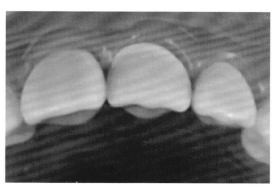

图 2-30　切端观

唇面预备

According to the method of the incisal 2/3 labial surface preparation, the same bur is parallel to the cervical 1/3 labial surface. According to the depth grooves, the tissue from the distal to mesial of the cervical 1/3 labial surface is removed. Take care not to damage the adjacent tooth. Then the cervical finish line on labial surface is prepared, which is placed at the gingival margin. The margin is 1.0mm wide and slight concave with round internal line angle, following the gingival edge in the shape of a scallop(Fig 2-27).

On the lateral view, the direction of the bur is parallel to the cervical 2/3 axial surface (Fig 2-28).

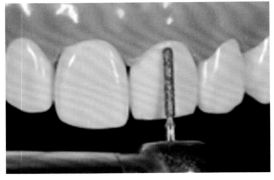
Fig 2-27　Prepare the cervical finish line

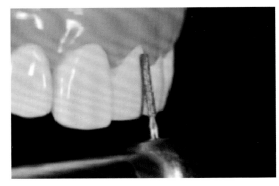
Fig 2-28　The lateral view

Tooth preparation of the labial surface is finished, the labial contour of which is the same as the natural tooth anatomical contour(Fig 2-29). The incisal 2/3 surface intersects smoothly with the cervical 1/3 surface. The preparation is extended to contact area as much as possible from the mesiodistal marginal ridge. Take care not to damage the adjacent tooth.

The incisal view of the finished labial surface(Fig 2-30).

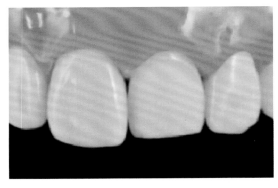
Fig 2-29　The labial preparation is finished

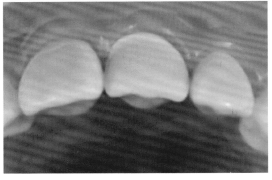
Fig 2-30　The incisal view

四、邻面预备

　　首先是打开邻接，邻面预备的要点：①切勿伤及邻牙；②近远中向的聚合度应控制在 2°～6°。使用细针状金刚砂车针沿与牙体长轴平行的方向从唇面远中边缘嵴切入（图 2-31），逐步穿透至腭侧面，此过程完全在预备牙牙体组织上进行，车针穿过腭侧后仍保留邻面牙体组织釉质薄片，避免伤及邻牙。

　　因前牙颈部是收窄的，故沿牙体长轴继续向根方预备（图 2-32），直至釉质薄片脱落，就可以完全打开远中邻接（图 2-33），使用相同方法打开近中邻接（图 2-34）。

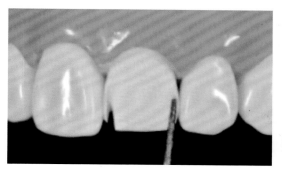

图 2-31　远中切 2/3 邻面预备

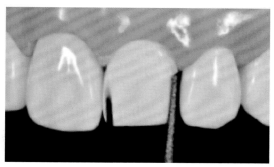

图 2-32　远中颈 1/3 邻面预备

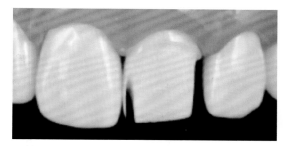

图 2-33　打开远中邻接

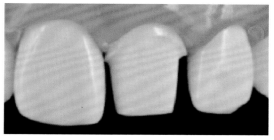

图 2-34　打开近中邻接

　　此时已消除了邻面接触区，然后换用直径 1.0mm 的圆头柱状金刚砂车针，在近远中邻面制备顺应龈乳头走行的颈部邻面边缘线（图 2-35），宽度为 1.0mm、平齐龈缘、内线角圆钝，并与唇面的边缘线移行过渡，预备时勿伤及邻牙。

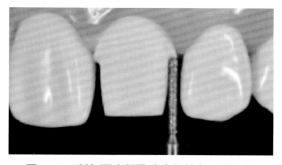

图 2-35　制备顺应龈乳头走行的邻面边缘线

4. Preparation of Proximal Surface

First, remove the contact area. The key points of the preparation are that ① do not damage the adjacent tooth, ② the convergence angle of mesial and distal surfaces should be kept at 2°-6°. The proximal reduction is performed with a fine needle-like diamond bur, which is parallel to the long axial of the tooth to sink into the tooth from the labial distal marginal ridge(Fig 2-31), and cuts through the palatal surface gradually. This process is performed on the prepared tooth tissue totally. In this sequence there are thin enamel chips remained in the proximal surface after the bur cutting through the palatal tooth, taking care not to damage the adjacent tooth.

Because the cervical part of the anterior tooth is narrowing, keep on preparing to root along the axial of the tooth(Fig 2-32). Until the enamel chips drop, the proximal contact is broken, then the proximal contact is broken(Fig 2-33). Remove the mesial contact by the same method(Fig 2-34).

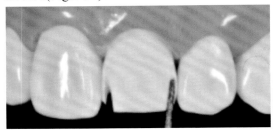

Fig 2-31　Prepare the incisal 2/3 distal proximal surface

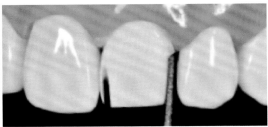

Fig 2-32　Prepare the cervical 1/3 distal proximal surface

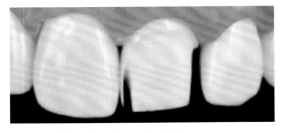

Fig 2-33　Open the distal contact

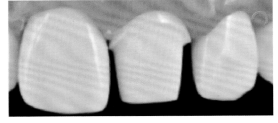

Fig 2-34　Open the mesial contact

The contact area is removed. Replace the bur by a 1.0mm diameter round-end cylindrical diamond to prepare a cervical margin line following the gingival papilla outline on the mesio-distal proximal surfaces(Fig 2-35). The cervical margin line is 1.0mm-wide and placed at the gingival margin with round internal line angle. The margin connects to the labial margin line, taking care not to damage the adjacent tooth.

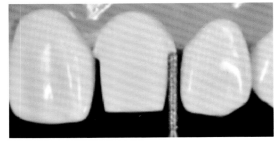

Fig 2-35　Prepare the line following the gingival papilla outline

邻面预备完成，消除了邻面倒凹，近远中邻面的聚合度应控制在 2°～6°（图 2-36）。

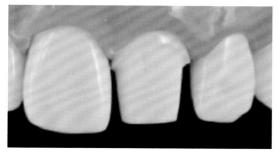

图 2-36　完成邻面预备

邻面预备

五、腭面预备

上中切牙腭侧面有几个重要的解剖结构：腭轴面、腭隆突及腭面边缘嵴，在前牙行使功能时有极其重要的作用。为了使最终修复体也能制作出相应的解剖结构，在预备时应保留这些解剖结构的轮廓及预备出足够的修复体空间。首先是腭轴面的预备，预备量为 1.0mm，使用直径 1.0mm 的圆头柱状车针切入腭轴面（图 2-37），方向与唇面颈 1/3 轴面平行，深度为 1.0mm，车针恰好完全没入，制备腭轴面的深度指示沟。近中面观，车针放置方向与唇面颈 1/3 轴面平行（图 2-38）。

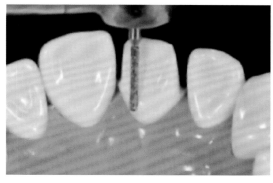

图 2-37　腭轴面深度指示沟预备

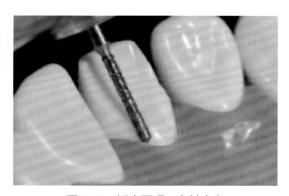

图 2-38　近中面观，车针方向

按照图 2-37 的方法完成腭轴面两条深度指示沟的预备（图 2-39）。

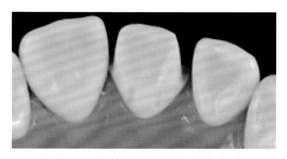

图 2-39　腭轴面两条深度指示沟完成

21

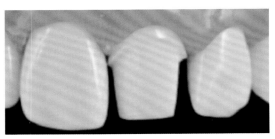

The preparation of the proximal surface is finished. The undercut area on the proximal surfaces is removed, and the taper of the mesial and distal proximal surfaces is 2°-6° (Fig 2-36).

Fig 2-36 The preparation of the proximal surface is finished

5. Preparation of Palatal Surface

The maxillary central incisor keeps several key anatomical structures, such as the palatal axial surface, the palatal protuberance, and the palatal marginal ridge, which play important role in anterior functional condition. To fabricate the corresponding anatomical structure on the restoration, whose contour should be kept and enough reduction should be prepared. First, prepare the palatal axial surface; the reduction is 1.0mm. A 1.0mm diameter round-end cylindrical diamond is used. The bur is sunk into the palatal axial surface(Fig 2-37), which is parallel to the cervical 1/3 labial surface. The depth is 1.0mm, making sure the diamond is inserted into the palatal axial surface depth orientation grooves to its full diameter. On the mesial view, the bur is parallel to the labial cervical 1/3 axial surface(Fig 2-38).

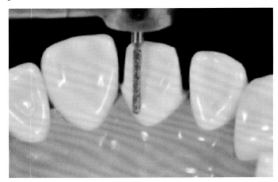

Fig 2-37 Prepare depth orientation grooves on palatal axial surface

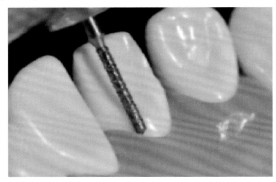

Fig 2-38 The mesial view of the bar direction

Two depth grooves on palatal axial surface are prepared as the method of Fig 2-37（Fig 2-39）.

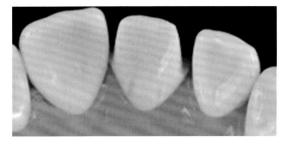

Fig 2-39 The preparation of two depth orientation grooves on palatal axial surface is finished

完成腭轴面深度指示沟后，使用同一车针沿腭轴面与唇面颈 1/3 轴面平行的方向，以深度指示沟为参考，按照腭轴面的解剖轮廓外形均匀磨除腭侧颈部远中到近中的牙体组织，避免伤及邻牙。颈部预备至平齐龈缘处，形成宽度为 0.5 ～ 0.8mm、内线角圆钝的颈部边缘线（图 2-40），并与邻面贯通，做到自然移行过渡。

在预备时，车针方向与唇面颈 1/3 轴面平行（图 2-41）。预备量约为 1.0mm，与唇面颈 1/3 轴面聚合度控制在 2° ～ 6°，形成制锁角，防止全冠旋转脱位，完成腭轴面预备（图 2-42）。

在完成腭轴面预备后，更换直径 2.0mm 的球形金刚砂车针在舌窝制备 3 ～ 4 个深度指示窝（图 2-43），深度为 1.0mm，相当于此车针的半径。

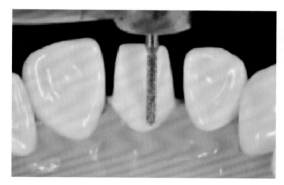

图 2-40　腭侧颈部边缘线预备

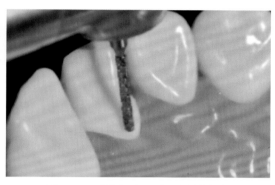

图 2-41　腭侧颈部预备时车针方向

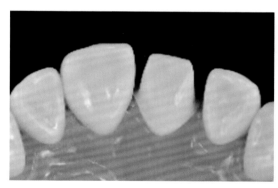

图 2-42　腭轴面预备完成

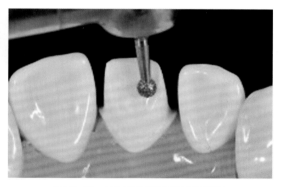

图 2-43　舌窝深度指示窝的预备

After the depth grooves on palatal axial surface are prepared, use the same bur along the palatal axial surface, parallel to the cervical 1/3 of the facial surface to remove the tissues evenly, which are between distal and mesial tissue on palatal cervical part following the contour of the palatal axial anatomical contour according to the depth grooves, taking care not to damage the adjacent tooth. The cervical finish line is placed at the gingival margin. The margin is 0.5-0.8mm wide with round internal line angle(Fig 2-40), and connects to the proximal surface naturally.

The bur is parallel to the cervical 1/3 of the labial surface(Fig 2-41) during the preparation process. The reduction is about 1.0mm, keeps a 2°-6° convergence with the labial cervical 1/3 axial surface to form a lock-angle; in case of rotating dislocation, the preparation of palatal axial surface is finished(Fig 2-42).

After the preparation of the palatal axial surface, replace the bur by 2.0mm diameter football shape diamond to make 3-4 depth fossa marks in lingual fossa(Fig 2-43). The depth is 1.0mm which is equal to a diameter of the bur.

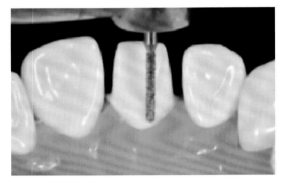

Fig 2-40   The preparation of the cervical finish line on palatal surface

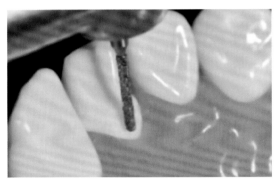

Fig 2-41   The direction of the bur when we prepare the palatal axial surface

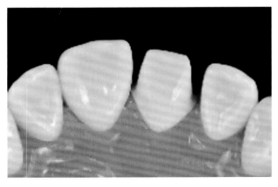

Fig 2-42   The palatal axial surface is prepared

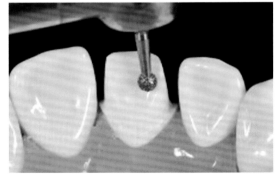

Fig 2-43   The depth fossae in lingual cingulum is prepared

此过程为防止球钻切入牙体组织过深，操作中车针柄应与牙长轴平行起到止动作用（图 2-44）。按照图 2-44 的方法在舌窝完成三个 1.0mm 的深度指示窝的预备（图 2-45）。

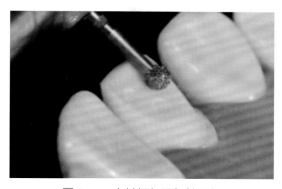

图 2-44　车针柄与牙长轴平行

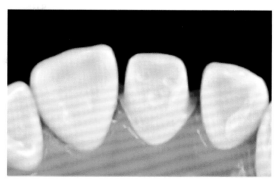

图 2-45　舌窝深度指示窝预备完成

然后换用橄榄球形金刚砂车针沿舌窝的解剖外形磨除深度指示窝之间的牙体组织（图 2-46）。此步骤预备量为 1.0mm，磨除范围包括两侧边缘嵴，并向根方越过舌隆突与舌轴壁贯通。预备时，橄榄球形金刚砂车针的放置方向平行于牙长轴方向（图 2-47）。预备完成后保留原舌窝的轮廓形态（图 2-48）。

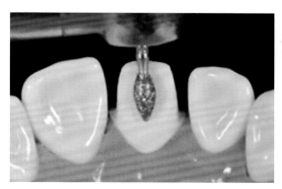

图 2-46　指示窝之间牙体组织的磨除

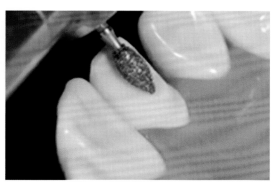

图 2-47　舌窝预备时车针的方向

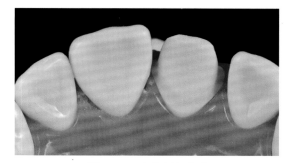

图 2-48　舌窝预备完成

腭侧面预备

In case of entering tissue too deep，the bur is parallel to the long axial of the tooth to limit moving(Fig 2-44). Three 1.0mm depth fossae in lingual fossa are prepared as methods of Fig 2-44 (Fig 2-45).

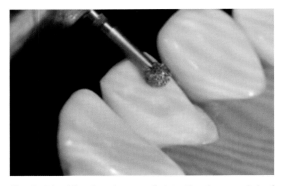

Fig 2-44　The bur is parallel to the long axial of the tooth

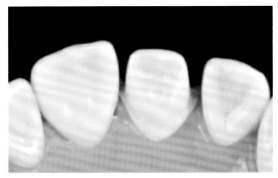

Fig 2-45　The preparation of the depth fossae on lingual fossa is finished

Replace the bur by the rugby shape diamond，remove the tissue between the depth fossae along the outline of the lingual cingulum(Fig 2-46). The reduction is 1.0mm，which covers the marginal ridge of both sides and connects to the lingual axial wall crossing the lingual protuberance towards the root. The bur is parallel to the long axial of the tooth(Fig 2-47). The finished preparation keeps the original cingulum concave shape (Fig 2-48).

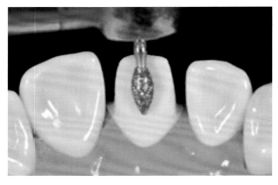

Fig 2-46　The tissue between the fossae is removed

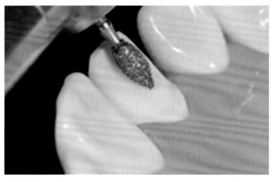

Fig 2-47　The direction of the bur in lingual cingulum in the process of preparation

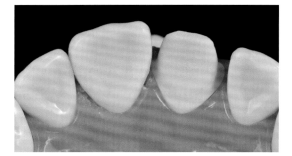

Fig 2-48　The preparation of lingual cingulum is finished

六、边缘修整，精修完成

在完成各个轴面及舌面窝的预备后，进行龈边缘的修整及精修与磨光。使用直径1.0mm的圆头柱状金刚砂车针修整唇面颈部边缘线（图2-49）、近远中邻面边缘线（图2-50）、腭侧颈部边缘线（图2-51），使其完全顺应龈缘走行，各轴面边缘线连续贯通、光滑一致，预备可采用排龈技术，避免伤及牙龈。

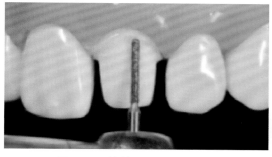

图2-49 修整唇面颈部边缘线

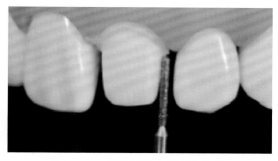

图2-50 修整近远中邻面边缘线

此后更换直径1.2mm的细粒度圆头柱状金刚砂车针，将各轴面、线角、轴角和面角修整圆钝并磨光（图2-52、图2-53），同时消除颈部边缘线飞边，预备时避免伤及牙龈。

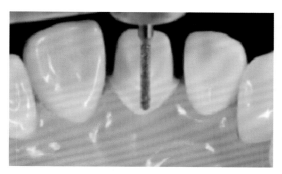

图2-51 修整腭侧颈部边缘线

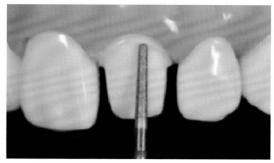

图2-52 磨光各轴面、线角、轴角和面角

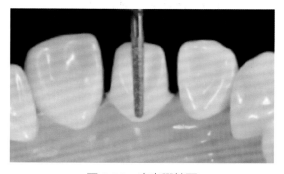

图2-53 磨光腭轴面

6. Margin Line is Prepared，and Fine Trimming Process is Finished

Trim，fine trim and polish the gingival margin line when the preparations of all axial surfaces and lingual fossa are finished. The labial(Fig 2-49)，mesiodistal(Fig 2-50)，palatal(Fig 2-51) cervical finish lines are trimmed by the 1.0mm diameter round-end cylindrical diamond following the direction of the gingival margin. Every line in axial surfaces connects to each other smoothly and uniformly. The preparation can adopt gingiva retraction technique. Take care not to damage the gingiva.

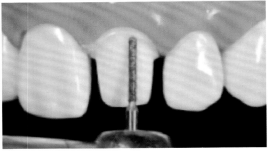

Fig 2-49　The cervical margin line on labial surface is finished

Fig 2-50　The distal and mesial proximal margin lines are trimmed

Replace the bur by a 1.2mm diameter fine-grained round-end cylindrical diamond to smooth and polish the axial surfaces，line angles，axial angles and plane angles(Fig 2-52，Fig 2-53). Remove the cervical margin line flash. Be careful not to damage the gingiva.

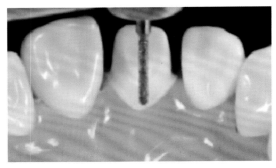

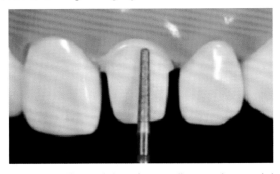

Fig 2-51　The palatal margin line is trimmed

Fig 2-52　The axial surfaces，line angles，axial angles and plane angles are polished

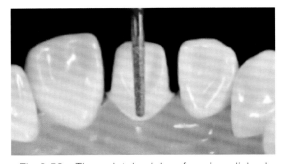

Fig 2-53　The palatal axial surface is polished

牙体缺损修复备牙过程图解

对于舌面窝，使用细粒度橄榄球形金刚砂车针将舌窝和线面角修整圆钝，磨光舌面（图 2-54）。

最后使用锐利的边缘修整器械修整预备体颈部边缘线，使之光滑、连续、完整（图 2-55 ～图 2-57）。

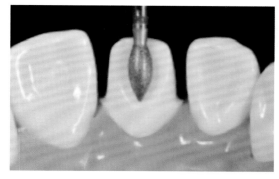

图 2-54　磨光舌窝和线面角

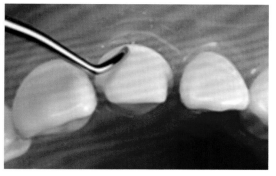

图 2-55　修整唇面颈部边缘线

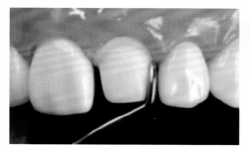

图 2-56　修整邻面边缘线

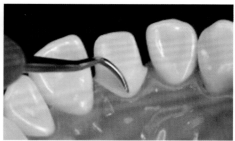

图 2-57　修整腭侧边缘线

边缘修整，精修完成

七、预备体检查

在完成所有的预备之后，对预备体做最后的检查，包括直视检查和 index 检查。完成的全瓷冠预备体唇面观（图 2-58）。

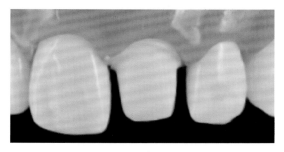

图 2-58　预备体唇面观

The fine-grained rugby shape diamond is used to trim the lingual fossa and the line angle，then polish the palatal surface(Fig 2-54).

The sharp fringe trimmer is used to trim the cervical margin line，so that the line is smooth，ontinuous，and complete(Fig 2-55-Fig 2-57).

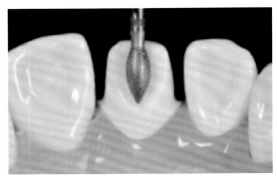

Fig 2-54　Polish the lingual fossa，line angle and plane angle

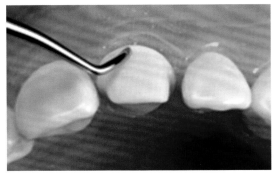

Fig 2-55　Trim the cervical margin line on labial surface

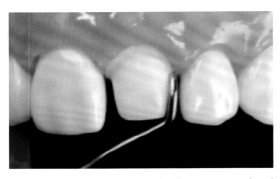

Fig 2-56　Trim the margin line on proximal surface

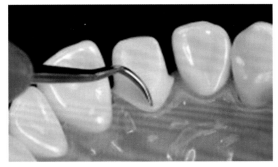

Fig 2-57　Trim the margin line on palatal surface

7. Check of the Tooth Preparation

Check the preparation finally after the process of tooth preparation through observation and the index. The labial view of the preparation for an all-ceramic crown(Fig 2-58).

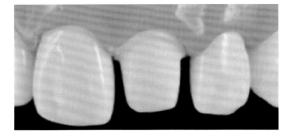

Fig 2-58　The labial view of the finished preparation

完成的预备体切端观，预备体呈圆三角形（图 2-59）。完成预备体腭面观预备后仍可见腭轴面、舌面窝及舌隆突等解剖轮廓外形（图 2-60）。

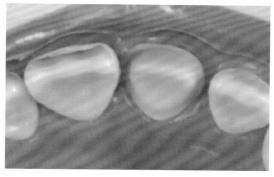

图 2-59　预备体切端观

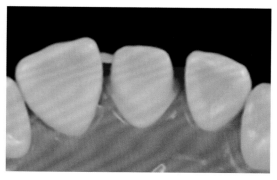

图 2-60　预备体腭面观

index-Ⅱ 戴入后见预备体轮廓外形近远中走向及切端与原牙平行一致（图 2-61）。戴入 index-Ⅰ 检查，完成的预备体唇面形态与原牙的解剖轮廓一致。使用牙周探针检查唇面切 2/3 的预备量为 1.4mm（图 2-62），检查颈部 1/3 的预备量为 1.0mm（图 2-63），从切端到颈部预备量逐步减小。

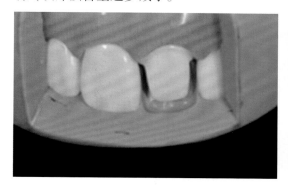

图 2-61　预备体轮廓与原牙一致

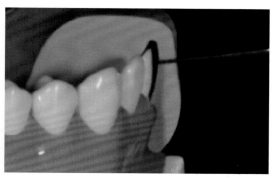

图 2-62　检查唇面切 2/3 的预备量

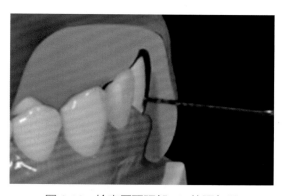

图 2-63　检查唇面颈部 1/3 的预备量

31

On the incisal view, the contour of the preparation is a circle triangle(Fig 2-59). On the lingual view, the preparation keeps the original anatomical contour including palatal axial surface, lingual fossa and lingual protuberance(Fig 2-60).

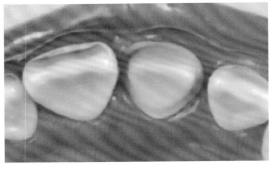

Fig 2-59　The incisal view of the preparation

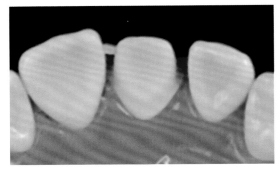

Fig 2-60　The palatal view of the preparation

The index-II is put into the mouth to check the contour of the preparation consistent in the uncut tooth following the incisal mesiodistal direction (Fig 2-61). The index-I is put into the mouth to check the contour of the preparation consistent in the uncut tooth on labial surface. The periodontal probe is used to check the 1.4mm-wide incisal 2/3 reduction (Fig 2-62) and the 1.0mm reduction on cervical 1/3 labial surface(Fig 2-63). The reduction of the labial is gradually decreased from the incisal edge to the cervical area.

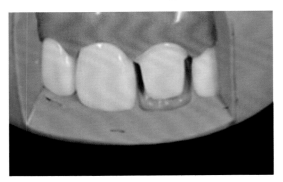

Fig 2-61　The preparation is consistent with the appearance of the uncut tooth

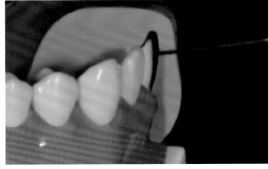

Fig 2-62　The reduction of incisal 2/3 labial surface is checked

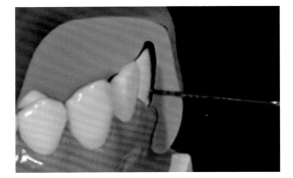

Fig 2-63　The reduction of cervical 1/3 labial surface is checked

预备体腭侧形态也与原牙的解剖轮廓一致，预备量为 1.0mm（图 2-64），切端预备量约为 2.0mm（图 2-65）。

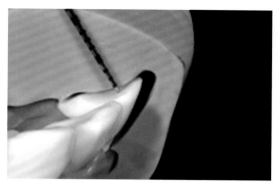
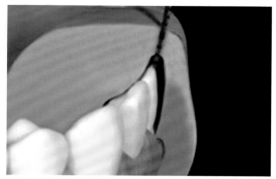

图 2-64　检查腭侧预备量　　　　　图 2-65　检查切端预备量

八、预备体展示

为了使读者更深刻地认识最终完成的规范上前牙全瓷冠牙体预备体的形态，我们将该牙粒从模型上摘下来观察：

牙体预备完成（唇面观），与原牙的解剖轮廓一致，边缘线（黄色线）走行与牙龈缘及釉牙骨质界（红色线）平行（图 2-66）。

牙体预备完成（腭面观），与原牙的解剖轮廓一致，边缘线（黄色线）走行与牙龈缘及釉牙骨质界（红色线）平行，绿色标记为舌轴面（图 2-67）。

牙体预备完成（近中邻面观），与原牙的解剖轮廓一致，边缘线（黄色线）走行与牙龈乳头及釉牙骨质界（红色线）平行（图 2-68）。

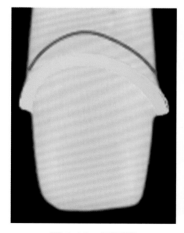
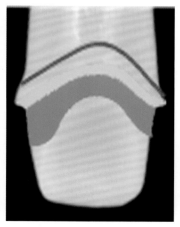
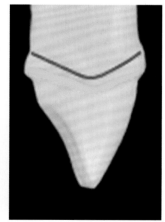

图 2-66　唇面观　　　　　图 2-67　腭面观　　　　　图 2-68　近中邻面观

The prepared palatal surface has the same anatomy contour with the original cingulum. The reduction of palatal surface is about 1.0mm(Fig 2-64). The reduction of the incisal edge is about 2.0mm(Fig 2-65).

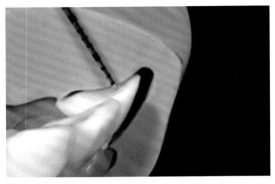 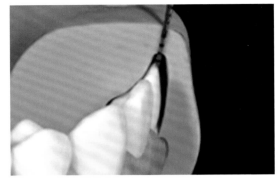

Fig 2-64   The reduction of palatal surface is checked   Fig 2-65   The reduction of incisal edge is checked

8. Display of the Tooth Preparation

In order to get a deeper insight into the final finished normative contour of the inferior incisal preparation，we pick the preparation out of the model.

The labial view of the finished preparation shows that the shape follows the general contours of the original tooth. The margin line(yellow line) follows the contour of the gingival tissue and cementum enamel junction(CEJ)(red line) (Fig 2-66).

The lingual view of the finished preparation shows that the shape follows the general contours of the original tooth. The margin line(yellow line) follows the contour of the gingival tissue and CEJ(red line). Green line is marked as the lingual-axial line(Fig 2-67).

The mesial view of the finished preparation shows that the shape follows the general contours of the original tooth. The margin line(yellow line) follows the contour of the gingival tissue and CEJ(red line) (Fig 2-68).

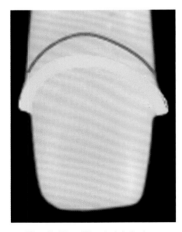 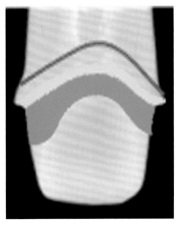 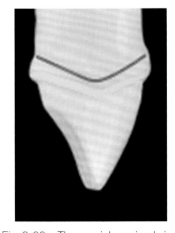

Fig 2-66   The labial view   Fig 2-67   The palatal view   Fig 2-68   The mesial proximal view

　　牙体预备完成远中邻面观（图 2-69），与原牙的解剖轮廓一致，边缘线（黄色线）走行与牙龈乳头及釉牙骨质界（红色线）平行。

　　牙体预备完成切端观（图 2-70），呈圆三角形，与原牙的解剖轮廓一致。

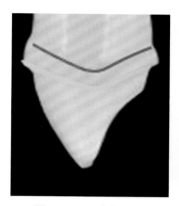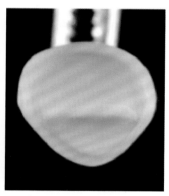

图 2-69　远中邻面观　　　　图 2-70　切端观

The distal view of the finished preparation(Fig 2-69). The shape follows the general contours of the original tooth. The margin line(yellow line) parallels the undulant papillae gingiva and CEJ (red line).

The incisal view of the finished preparation(Fig 2-70). The shape is rounded triangular, which follows the general contours of the original tooth.

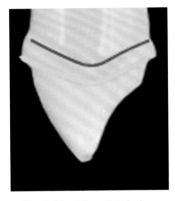 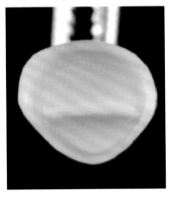

Fig 2-69　The distal view　　　Fig 2-70　The incisal view

第三章　前牙瓷贴面牙体预备

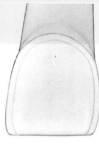

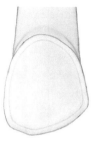

　　贴面是在微量磨牙或少量磨牙的情况下，应用粘接技术，将复合树脂、瓷等修复材料覆盖在表面缺损患牙、着色牙、变色牙或畸形牙等上，用以恢复牙体正常形态或改善其色泽的一种修复方法。

　　经典的全瓷贴面牙体预备的设计可以分为三型：开窗型（window type）、对接型（butt-joint type）和包绕型（overlap type）。对接型和包绕型在切端均有修复体覆盖，贴面在对刃切割等功能状态时承受的是压应力，符合瓷材料耐压不抗拉的特性，有利于预防瓷修复体损坏，延长修复体寿命。另外，这种设计还能帮助贴面准确就位和有效粘接，并可减少贴面内的应力集中。当切端需要重塑时，多采用对接型贴面预备；如果切端有足够的牙体组织厚度，可以采用包绕型贴面预备，当切端不需要重塑时，则建议采用开窗型贴面预备。

　　本章就此三种经典的贴面预备形式，分别以 21 牙和 23 牙为例进行图文视听介绍。

Chapter 3　Anterior Tooth Preparation for Veneer

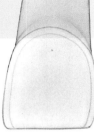

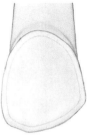

With grinding traces or a small amount of tooth, the veneer is a restoring method with the binding technology to cover the defected tooth, shaded tooth, discolored tooth or distorted tooth by restoration materials such as composite resin and ceramic, which aims at modifying the shape and color of the tooth.

The classic preparation design of the all-ceramic veneer is classified into three different types: window type, butt-joint type and overlap type. The latter two types of restorations cover the incisal edge, which bear the compressive force in the function of edge-to-edge and incision in line with the feature of pressure resistant and tension intolerance. In this way, it may prevent the damage of ceramic restoration to extend its life. Besides, the design can make the veneer insert and attach accurately and distribute occlusal forces over a larger surface area. When we reshape the incisal edge, we apply the butt-joint type more. If the incisal tissue is thick enough, the overlap type can be chosen. When the incisal edge do not need to be reshaped, we recommend to adopt the window type.

The chapter takes the 21 and 23 tooth as examples describing these three classic veener preparation designs.

第一节　对接型、包绕型瓷贴面牙体预备

对接型、包绕型瓷贴面预备流程及牙体预备量见图 3-1。

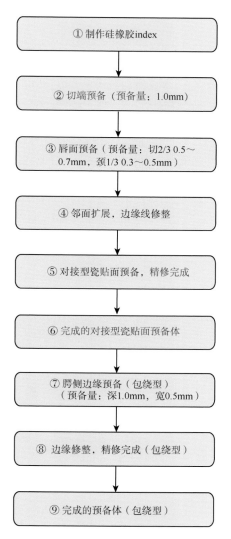

① 制作硅橡胶 index

② 切端预备（预备量：1.0mm）

③ 唇面预备（预备量：切 2/3 0.5～0.7mm，颈 1/3 0.3～0.5mm）

④ 邻面扩展，边缘线修整

⑤ 对接型瓷贴面预备，精修完成

⑥ 完成的对接型瓷贴面预备体

⑦ 腭侧边缘预备（包绕型）（预备量：深 1.0mm，宽 0.5mm）

⑧ 边缘修整，精修完成（包绕型）

⑨ 完成的预备体（包绕型）

图 3-1　对接型、包绕型瓷贴面预备流程及牙体预备量

Section 1 Porcelain Veneer Preparation of Anterior Tooth（Butt-Joint Type and Overlap Type）

The process of butt-joint type and overlap type veneer preparations and the tooth reduction are shown in Fig 3-1.

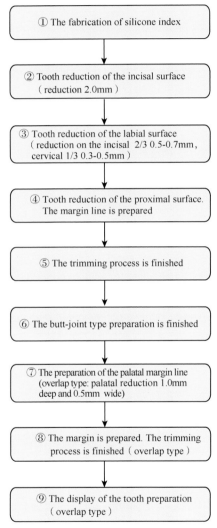

① The fabrication of silicone index

② Tooth reduction of the incisal surface
（reduction 2.0mm）

③ Tooth reduction of the labial surface
（reduction on the incisal 2/3 0.5-0.7mm,
cervical 1/3 0.3-0.5mm）

④ Tooth reduction of the proximal surface.
The margin line is prepared

⑤ The trimming process is finished

⑥ The butt-joint type preparation is finished

⑦ The preparation of the palatal margin line
(overlap type: palatal reduction 1.0mm
deep and 0.5mm wide)

⑧ The margin is prepared. The trimming
process is finished（overlap type）

⑨ The display of the tooth preparation
（overlap type）

Fig 3-1　The process and reduction of the butt-joint type and overlap type veneer preparations

一、制作硅橡胶 index

此部分同第二章第一部分制作硅橡胶 index 的方法，只需要制作 index-Ⅰ（见图 2-2、图 2-3）。

二、切端预备

对于对接型贴面及包绕型贴面，患牙的切端是需要重塑的，牙体预备也从切端开始。使用末端直径 1.0mm 的圆头锥状金刚砂车针，沿 21 牙原切端磨耗斜面的方向切入牙体组织。预备切端深度指示沟，深度约 1.0mm，车针恰好没入，预备至少两个深度指示沟（图 3-2）。使用同一车针沿原来切端的近远中走行，磨除远中切角到远中深度指示沟之间的牙体组织，在磨除远中切角时避免伤及邻牙（图 3-3）。磨除后的唇面观（图 3-4）、切端观（图 3-5）。

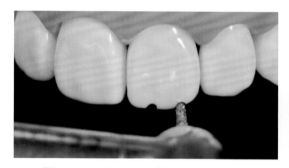

图 3-2　深度 1.0mm 的两个深度指示沟

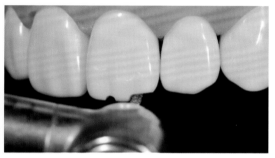

图 3-3　磨除远中切角到远中深度指示沟之间的牙体组织

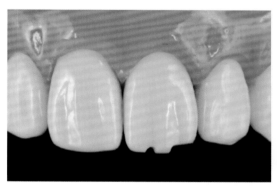

图 3-4　唇面观

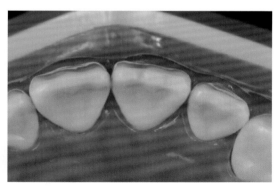

图 3-5　切端观

1. Fabrication of Silicone Index

Fabricate the same silicone index as methods of part one on chapter 2，it just need to make index-Ⅰ (Fig 2-2，Fig 2-3).

2. Preparation of Incisal Edge

As for butt-joint type and overlap type veneers，we except the incisal edge to be reshape. The preparation process begins at the incisal edge. Use a 1.0mm diameter round-end tapered diamond bur. This bur is sunk into tissue along the inclination of 21 tooth incisal wear facets. Then prepare the incisal edge depth orientation grooves，the depth of the grooves is 1.0mm. The bur is sunk into the incisal edge，where at least two grooves are made(Fig 3-2). The same bur is extended from distal depth orientation groove to distal-incisal angle along the mesial distal direction of the incisal edge，taking care not to damage the adjacent tooth when removing the distal-incisal angle(Fig 3-3).The labial view after removing(Fig 3-4). The incisal view(Fig 3-5).

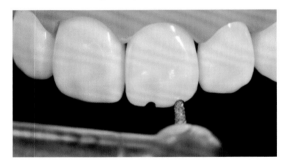

Fig 3-2　Two incisal depth orientation grooves are 1.0mm deep

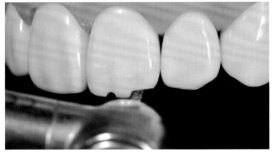

Fig 3-3　Remove tissue from distal-incisal angle to distal depth orientation groove

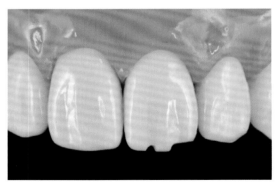

Fig 3-4　The labial view

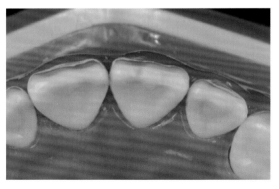

Fig 3-5　The incisal view

　　按照上述方法依次磨除切端近中边缘嵴到远中定深沟之间的牙体组织（图 3-6）。预备后的切端近远中走行顺应原来的切端走行（图 3-7），唇腭向走行与原来的磨耗斜面平行（图 3-8、图 3-9）。

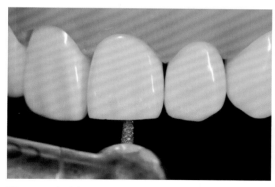

图 3-6　磨除切端近中边缘嵴到远中定深沟之间的牙体组织

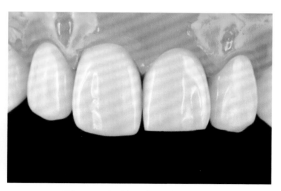

图 3-7　切端预备后的唇面观

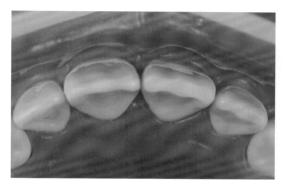

图 3-8　切端预备后的切端观

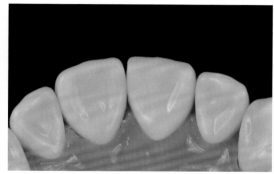

图 3-9　切端预备后的腭侧观

对接型切端预备

三、唇面预备

　　瓷贴面基牙唇面的预备须按照天然上前牙唇面的解剖特点分为切 2/3 及颈 1/3 两个轴面预备。首先是切 2/3 的唇面深度指示沟的预备。上前牙唇面切 2/3 的釉质可达 1.0mm 以上的厚度，为了实现瓷贴面更加生动的美学效果，在唇面切 2/3 预备 0.5mm 的深度指示沟。使用刃深 0.5mm 的深度指示车针，在唇面切 1/3 预备一条深度指示沟，车针刃部完全没入，深约 0.5mm（图 3-10）。车针放置方向：车针柄与切 2/3 轴面平行，防止车针切入牙体组织过深（图 3-11）。切 1/3 深度指示沟预备完成（唇面观如图 3-12，近中面观如图 3-13）。

The remaining tissue between the mesial marginal ridge and distal depth groove of incisal is removed gradually(Fig 3-6). The prepared incisal mesiodistal direction parallels the former incisal edge(Fig 3-7)，and labial-palatal direction parallels the original wear facet(Fig 3-8， Fig 3-9).

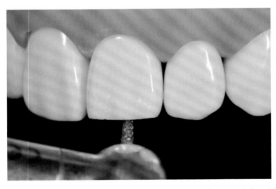

Fig 3-6 The tissue between the mesial ridge and distal depth orientation grooves of incisal edge is removed

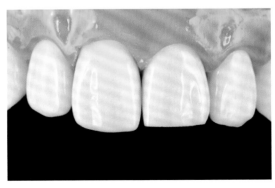

Fig 3-7 The labial view of the incisal edge after reduction

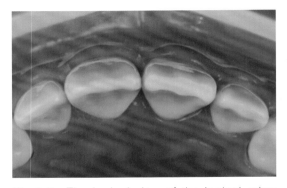

Fig 3-8 The incisal view of the incisal edge after reduction

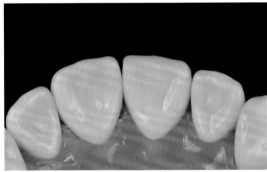

Fig 3-9 The palatal view of the incisal edge after reduction

3. Preparation of Labial Surface

According to the natural maxillary anterior anatomical feature，porcelain veneer preparation of the labial surface is separated by two parts：incisal 2/3 and cervical 1/3 axial surfaces. First，prepare the depth grooves on incisal 2/3 labial surface. The thickness of the incisal 2/3 labial surface enamel is above 1.0mm. To achieve better esthetics effect of the veneer，0.5mm deep depth grooves on incisal 2/3 labial surface are prepared. Use the bur by one with 0.5mm wide blade to make a depth groove on the incisal 1/3 labial surface. The bur is sunk into the tooth. The groove is 0.5mm deep(Fig 3-10). The bur is parallel to the incisal 2/3 axial surface (Fig 3-11). Then the preparation of incisal 1/3 depth grooves is finished(the labial view as shown in Fig 3-12，the mesial view as shown in Fig 3-13).

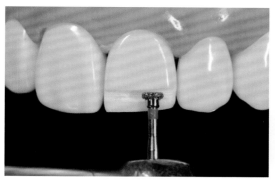

图 3-10　唇面切 1/3 0.5mm 深度指示沟的预备

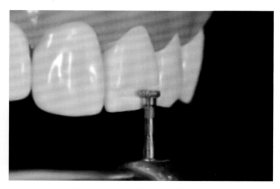

图 3-11　车针的放置方向

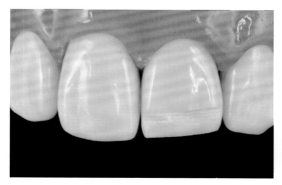

图 3-12　唇面观

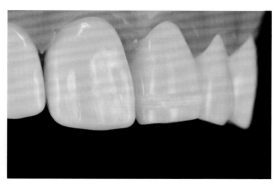

图 3-13　近中面观

　　使用相同的方法，在唇面中 1/3 预备第二条深 0.5mm 的深度指示沟（图 3-14）。车针放置时车针柄与切 2/3 轴面平行一致（图 3-15）。切 2/3 轴面深度指示沟完成（图 3-16、图 3-17）。

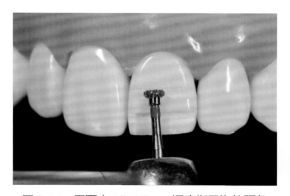

图 3-14　唇面中 1/3 0.5mm 深度指示沟的预备

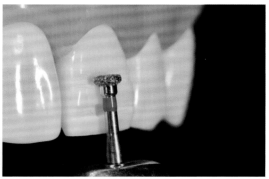

图 3-15　车针的放置方向

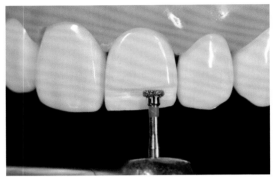

Fig 3-10 Preparing cervical 1/3 depth orientation groove with a depth of 0.5mm

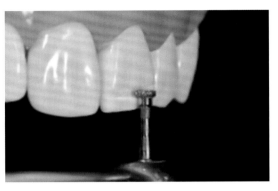

Fig 3-11 The direction of the bur

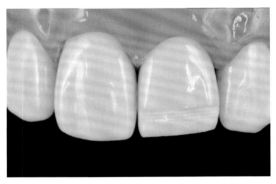

Fig 3-12 The labial view

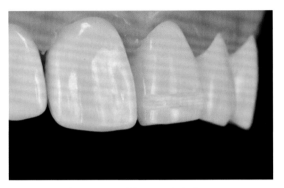

Fig 3-13 The mesial view

Prepare the second 0.5mm depth orientation groove on the middle 1/3 labial surface in the same way(Fig 3-14). The bur is parallel to the incisal 2/3 axial surface (Fig 3-15). The preparation of incisal 2/3 axial grooves is finished(Fig 3-16，Fig 3-17).

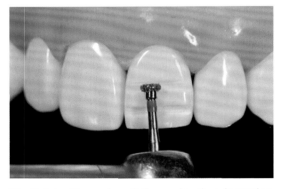

Fig 3-14 Preparing 0.5mm depth orientation groove on middle 1/3 labial surface

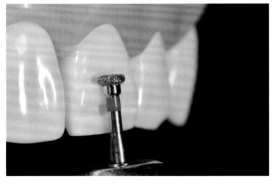

Fig 3-15 The direction of the bur

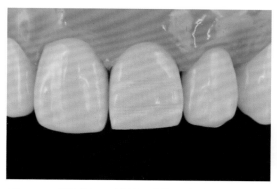

图 3-16 唇面切 2/3 轴面深度指示沟完成，唇面观

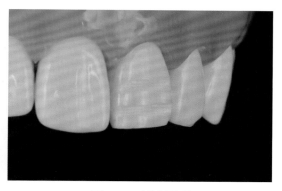

图 3-17 近中面观

在完成唇面切 2/3 两条 0.5mm 的深度指示沟后，更换刃深 0.3mm 的深度指示车针，在唇面颈 1/3 预备一条深约 0.3mm 的深度指示沟，车针刃部完全没入（图 3-18）。车针放置方向：车针柄与颈 1/3 轴面平行，防止车针切入牙体组织过深（图 3-19）。唇面深度指示沟预备完成后，在指示沟底使用马克笔涂上颜色标记（唇面观图 3-20、近中面观图 3-21）。

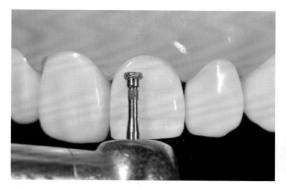

图 3-18 唇面颈 1/3 一条深约 0.3mm 的深度指示
　　　　 沟的预备

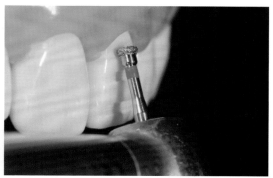

图 3-19 车针放置的方向

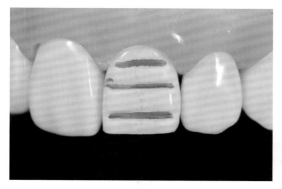

图 3-20 颜色标记唇面观

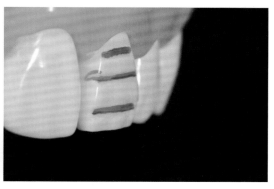

图 3-21 颜色标记近中面观

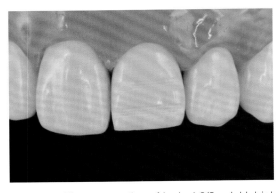

Fig 3-16　The preparation of incisal 2/3 axial labial surface depth orientation grooves is finished on the labial view

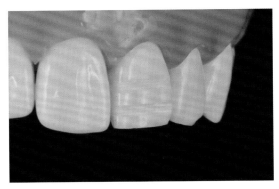

Fig 3-17　The mesial view

When the two 0.5mm deep incisal 2/3 depth grooves preparations are finished, the bur is replaced by a 0.3mm diameter round-end diamond depth cut bur. The bur is sunk into the cervical 1/3 on labial surface to make an approximate 0.3mm depth orientation groove(Fig 3-18). The direction of the bur: the bur maintains parallelism to the cervical 1/3 of the axial surface(Fig 3-19). When the preparation of the labial depth orientation grooves is finished, color the bottom of the depth orientation grooves for marking(the labial view as shown in Fig 3-20，the mesial view as shown in Fig 3-21).

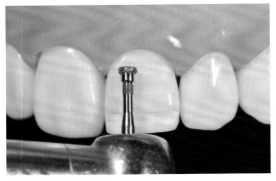

Fig 3-18　Preparing a 0.3mm depth orientation groove on cervical 1/3 labial surface

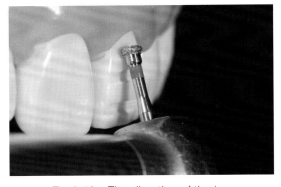

Fig 3-19　The direction of the bur

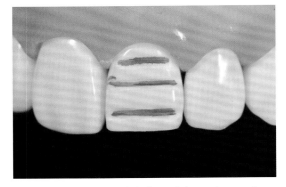

Fig 3-20　The labial view of the color mark

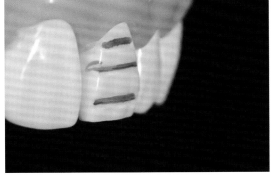

Fig 3-21　The mesial view of the color mark

　　唇面预备完成不同深度的指示沟后，开始进入到唇面深度指示沟间牙体组织的磨除过程。仍然按照唇面切 2/3 与颈 1/3 两个轴面分别预备，首先是唇面切 2/3 的预备。更换末端直径 1.0mm 的圆头锥状金刚砂车针，车针沿与唇面切 2/3 轴面平行的方向，参照深度指示沟的深度，磨除唇面切 2/3 远中边缘嵴到近中边缘嵴的牙体组织（图 3-22），预备时避免伤及邻牙。车针放置方向：车针柄与唇面切 2/3 轴面平行（图 3-23）。唇面切 2/3 轴面深度指示沟之间牙体组织初步磨除完成（图 3-24、图 3-25），沟底部的颜色标记不能完全被磨除，这样可以有效防止预备过量。

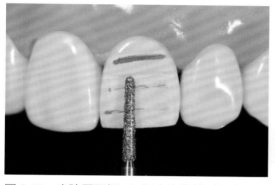

图 3-22　磨除唇面切 2/3 远中边缘嵴到近中边缘嵴的牙体组织

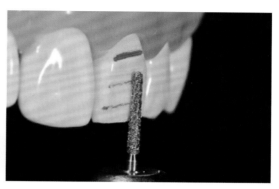

图 3-23　车针放置的方向

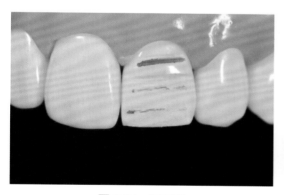

图 3-24　唇面观

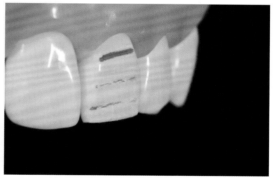

图 3-25　近中面观

　　使用同一车针沿与唇面颈 1/3 轴面平行的方向，按照深度指示沟的深度，磨除颈 1/3 远中到近中边缘嵴之间的牙体组织（图 3-26），颈部预备至平齐龈缘处，形成 0.3～0.4mm 宽、内线角圆钝的颈部边缘线。车针放置方向：车针柄与颈 1/3 轴面平行（图 3-27）。预备后的唇面与原牙解剖轮廓平行。预备量：切 2/3 为 0.5～0.7mm，颈 1/3 为 0.3～0.5mm，初步预备完成时深度指示沟底的颜色标记不完全被磨除（图 3-28），以防止牙体预备过量暴露过多的牙本质，唇面预备后仍保留上中切牙唇面两个轴面相交的解剖外形（图 3-29）。

The tissue between depth grooves is removed after the fabrication of the grooves. This process can be separated by two parts: incisal 2/3 and cervical 1/3 labial surface. First step is to prepare the former one. Replace the bur by a 1.0mm diameter round-end tapered diamond. The bur parallels the incisal 2/3 labial surface. The tissue between mesial and distal marginal ridge on the incisal 2/3 labial surface is removed according to the depth grooves(Fig 3-22). Be careful not to damage the adjacent tooth. The direction of the bur: the bur is parallel to the incisal 2/3 axial surface (Fig 3-23). The primary preparation of tissue between the depth grooves on the incisal 2/3 axial part on labial surface finished(the labial view as shown in Fig 3-24，the mesial view as shown in Fig 3-25). The color mark on the bottom of the grooves can not be removed completely in case of preparing too much.

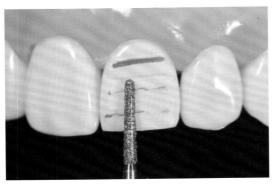

Fig 3-22　Remove the tissue between distal marginal ridge and mesial marginal ridge on labial incisal 2/3 surface

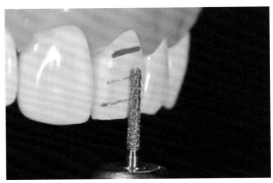

Fig 3-23　The direction of the bur

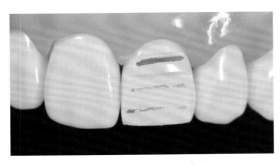

Fig 3-24　The labial view

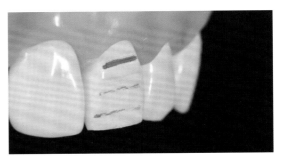

Fig 3-25　The mesial view

Use the same bur which parallels to the cervical 1/3 axial surface，remove the tissue between the mesial and distal marginal ridge on the cervical 1/3 labial surface according to the depth orientation grooves(Fig 3-26). The cervical tissue is prepared at the level of gingival margin，which forms 0.3-0.4mm wide cervical margin line with round internal corner. The direction of the bur: the bur is parallel to the cervical 1/3 surface(Fig 3-27). The labial surface of the prepared tooth is parallel to the anatomical contour of the original tooth. The reduction of the incisal 2/3 surface is 0.5-0.7mm，and the cervical 1/3 is 0.3-0.5mm. The color mark on the bottom of the depth grooves is not removed totally (Fig 3-28)，in case that the tooth is prepared too much to expose the dentin. After labial preparation，the anatomical contour of two axial surface on labial surface intersecting with each other is kept (Fig 3-29).

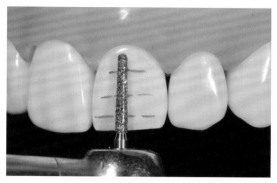

图 3-26　磨除唇面颈 1/3 远中到近中边缘嵴之间的牙体组织

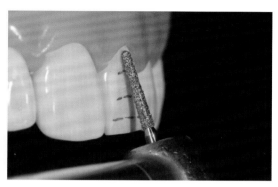

图 3-27　车针放置方向

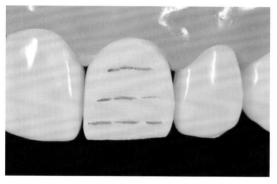

图 3-28　预备后的唇面与原牙解剖轮廓平行

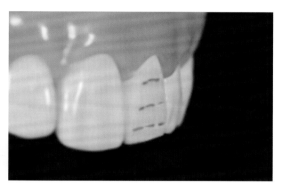

图 3-29　唇面预备完成，近中面观

四、邻面扩展，边缘线修整

贴面预备体的邻面边缘线多位于非自洁区，预备体可尽量向邻接区扩展，最大可进入邻接区的一半，但不能向腭侧突破邻接区，这样做可以有效将贴面修复体与基牙的边缘线隐藏起来，达到美观的效果。邻面预备首先是邻面边缘线的扩展，更换末端直径0.8mm 的圆头锥状金刚砂车针，从预备体唇面颈部边缘线开始分别向近远中邻面边缘扩展（图 3-30）。在龈外展隙处尽量向舌侧扩

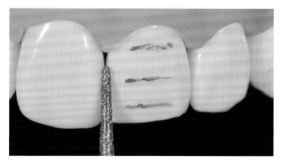

图 3-30　从预备体唇面向邻面扩展

展，使边缘线进入非自洁区，在邻接区尽量向腭侧扩展，但不完全破坏接触点，形成近远中 0.4 ~ 0.5mm 宽的边缘线，预备时为避免伤及邻牙，车针可翘起与轴面呈 30° ~ 45°（图 3-31），预备完成的邻面边缘线均位于非自洁区。

51

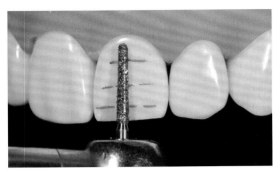

Fig 3-26　Remove tissue between mesial and distal marginal ridge on cervical 1/3 labial surface

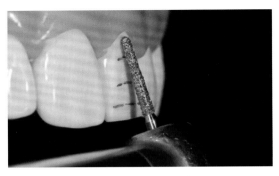

Fig 3-27　The direction of the bur

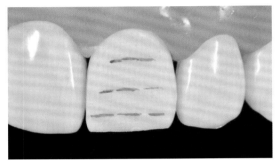

Fig 3-28　The labial surface of the prepared tooth is parallel to the anatomical contour of the original tooth

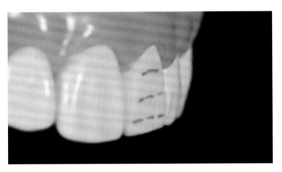

Fig 3-29　The labial preparation is finished on the mesial view

4. Preparation of Proximal Surface and Margin Line

The proximal finish line locates in the self-cleaning area mostly. Try to extend to contact area as much as possible, which can reach to the half part of the connecting area without crossing the contact point, so that the margin line of the restoration and abutment can be hidden to achieve esthetics effect. Firstly, extend the proximal finish line, replace the bur by a 0.8mm diameter round-end tapered diamond. The margin line is extended from labial cervical margin line to the mesiodistal proximal surface(Fig 3-30). Try to extend to lingual side in the gingival embrasure, so that the margin line enters the nonself-cleaning area, extends to palatal side on the contact area without damage to the contact point, which forms a 0.4-0.5mm wide mesiodistal margin line. Be careful not to damage the adjacent tooth. The bur is positioned at a 30°-45° inclination with the axial surface. The finish line locates in self-cleaning area(Fig 3-31).

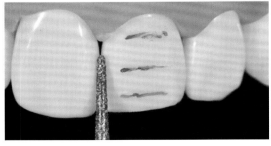

Fig 3-30　Extend from labial surface to the proximal surface

邻面预备完成的唇面观（图 3-32）。近中面观（图 3-33）邻面边缘线不被暴露出来。

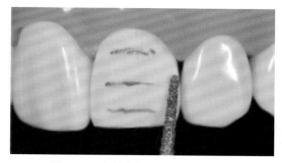

图 3-31　车针与轴面呈 30°～45°

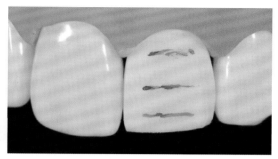

图 3-32　邻面预备完成，唇面观

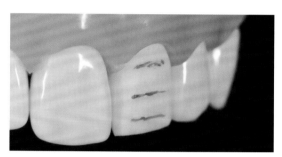

图 3-33　邻面预备完成，近中面观

五、精修完成

此步仅做精修与磨光，不再对预备体做更多的磨除。临床上，贴面更多的是依靠釉质粘接来提供固位力，预备体表面的过度抛光对于粘接是不利因素，但为了获得更加清晰准确的印模，预备体需要进行适度的磨光，使轴面光滑，边缘线清晰，点、线、面、角圆钝光滑，此过程推荐使用排龈技术。

精修时使用细粒度的末端直径 1.0mm 的圆头锥状金刚砂车针，将预备体唇面沿切 2/3 轴面（图 3-34）、颈 1/3 轴面（图 3-35）、唇面近中边缘线（图 3-36）、唇面颈部边缘线磨光（图 3-37），唇面远中边缘线（图 3-38）分别磨光，并消除边缘线飞边。

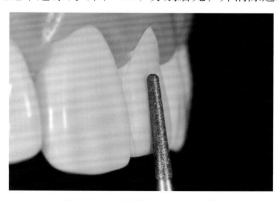

图 3-34　唇面切 2/3 轴面磨光

On labial view, the preparation of proximal surface is finished(Fig 3-32). On the mesial view, the proximal margin line is not exposed(Fig 3-33).

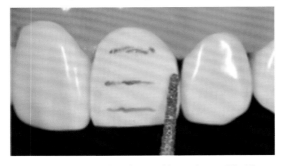

Fig 3-31   The bur is positioned at a 30-45 degrees inclination with the axial surface

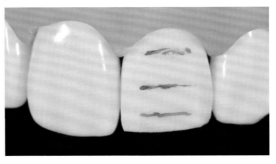

Fig 3-32   The labial view after the preparation of proximal surface

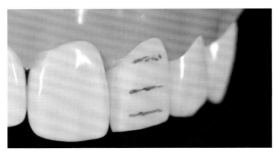

Fig 3-33   The mesial view after the preparation of proximal surface

5. Fine Trimming Process is Finished

The preparation needs to be trimmed and polished merely without reduction anymore. The retention of the veneer derives more from enamel attachment clinically. To polish excessively on the preparation surface is a negative factor. However, in order to get the impression more accurately, preparation needs to be polished moderately, which makes the axial surface smooth, the finish line clear and all points rounded and smooth. This process is recommended to perform gingival retraction.

The trimming process uses a 1.0mm diameter fine-grained round-end tapered diamond. Polish the incisal 2/3 of the axial surface(Fig 3-34), the cervical 1/3 of labial surface(Fig 3-35), the mesial margin line on labial surface(Fig 3-36), the cervical margin line(Fig 3-37) and the distal margin line on labial surface(Fig 3-38) separately, remove the flash of the margin line.

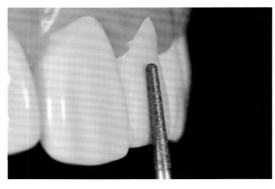

Fig 3-34   Polish the incisal 2/3 axial surface

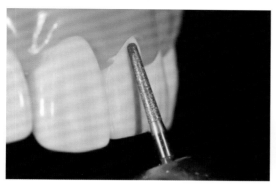

图 3-35　唇面颈 1/3 轴面磨光

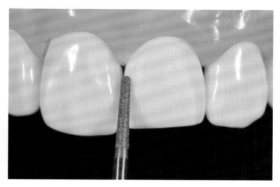

图 3-36　近中边缘线磨光，消除飞边

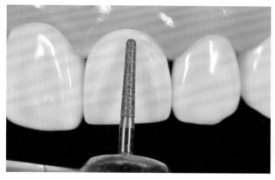

图 3-37　颈部边缘线磨光，消除飞边

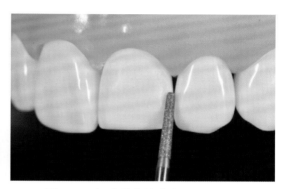

图 3-38　远中边缘线磨光，消除飞边

为了获得更加清晰、准确的边缘线，保证修复体与基牙的边缘适合性，可以使用锐利的边缘修整器械修整边缘线，使整个边缘线光滑、连续（图 3-39）。

唇 面、邻 面 预备与精修

对接型边缘修整

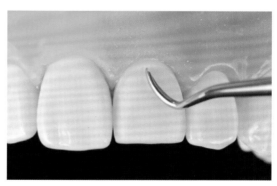

图 3-39　使用锐利的边缘修整器械修整边缘线

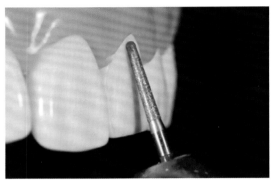

Fig 3-35　Polish the cervical 1/3 axial surface

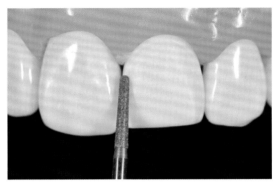

Fig 3-36　Polish the mesial margin line and
remove the flash

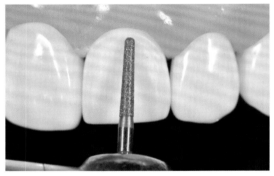

Fig 3-37　Polish the cervical margin line and
remove the flash

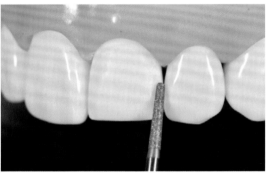

Fig 3-38　Polish the distal margin line and
remove the flash

　　To get the margin line more accurate for keeping the restoration and the preparation more dense，trim the margin line by sharp fringe trimmer，make the margin line smooth and continuous(Fig 3-39).

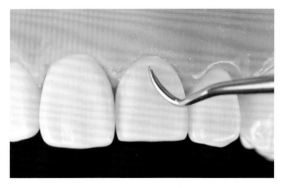

Fig 3-39　Trim the margin line by sharp trimmer

　　戴入 index-I，使用牙周探针检查可见唇面切 2/3 预备量为 0.5 ～ 0.7mm（图 3-40）。颈 1/3 预备量为 0.3 ～ 0.5mm（图 3-41）。切端预备量为 1.0mm（图 3-42）。精修完成的对接型贴面预备体唇面观见图 3-43、切端观见图 3-44、近中面观见图 3-45、远中面观见图 3-46，轴面光滑、线角、面角圆钝，边缘线清晰，仍保留了上中切牙原有的解剖轮廓外形。

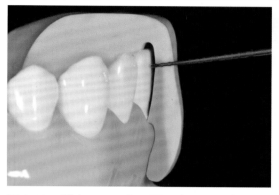

图 3-40　戴入 index-I，唇面切 2/3 预备量为 0.5 ～ 0.7mm

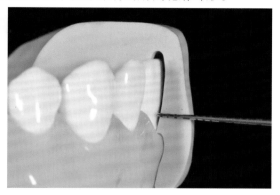

图 3-41　颈 1/3 预备量为 0.3 ～ 0.5mm

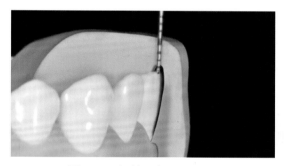

图 3-42　切端预备量 1.0mm

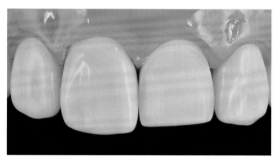

图 3-43　精修完成，唇面观

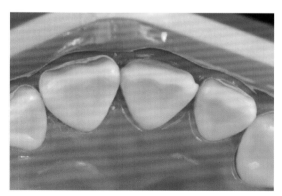

图 3-44　精修完成，切端观

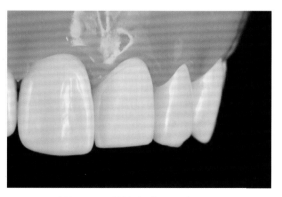

图 3-45　精修完成，近中面观

After putting the index-Ⅰ into the mouth，it shows the 0.5-0.7mm reduction of the incisal 2/3 of the labial surface with the periodontal probe(Fig 3-40)，the 0.3-0.5mm reduction of the cervical 1/3 of the labial surface(Fig 3-41)，and the 1.0mm reduction of the incisal edge (Fig 3-42). The finished butt-joint type veneer preparation is shown on the labial view as Fig 3-43，the incisal view as Fig 3-44，the mesial view as Fig 3-45，the distal view as Fig 3-46. All axial surfaces are smooth，the line angles and the plane angles are rounded，the margin line is clear. And the preparation keeps the anatomical contour of the original tooth.

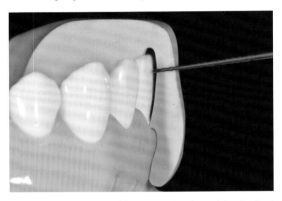

Fig 3-40　The index-Ⅰ, the reduction of the incisal 2/3 labial surface is 0.5-0.7mm

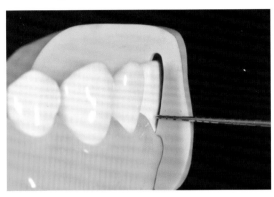

Fig 3-41　The 0.3-0.5mm reduction of the cervical 1/3 labial surface

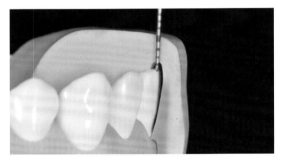

Fig 3-42　The 1.0mm reduction of the incisal edge

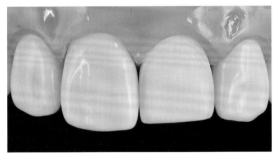

Fig 3-43　The trimming process is finished on the labial view

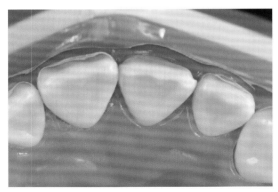

Fig 3-44　The trimming process is finished on the incisal view

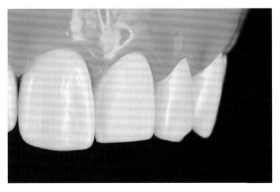

Fig 3-45　The trimming process is finished on the mesial view

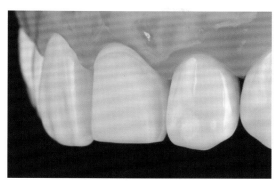

图 3-46　精修完成，远中面观

六、对接型瓷贴面预备体完成

完成的对接型瓷贴面预备体唇面观（图 3-47），切端观（图 3-48）。预备体表面光滑、平整、圆钝。

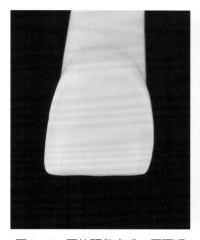

图 3-47　牙体预备完成，唇面观

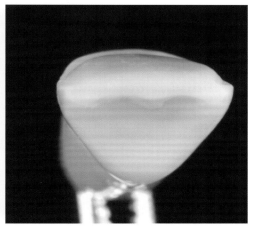

图 3-48　牙体预备完成，切端观

七、腭侧边缘预备（包绕型）

在完成的对接型贴面的基础上，增加预备腭侧的包绕形态，完成包绕型瓷贴面的牙体预备。换用末端直径 1.0mm 的圆头锥状金刚砂车针，在完成的对接型瓷贴面预备体切端腭侧面，预备出深度 1.0mm、宽度 0.5mm 的腭侧边缘线，须离开咬合接触区至少 1.0mm（图 3-49），咬合接触区或者接触线可以位于健康的牙体组织上，也可以落在修复体上，但不能落在修复体边缘线上。腭侧边缘线在近远中绕过切角与唇面近远中边缘线相延续且自然移行（图 3-50）。

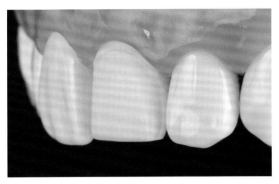

Fig 3-46　The trimming process is finished on the distal view

6. Preparation of Butt-Joint Type Porcelain Veneer is Finished

The labial view(Fig 3-47)，and the incisal view(Fig 3-48) of the finished preparation of butt-joint type porcelain veneer are shown. The preparation surface is smooth，flat and round.

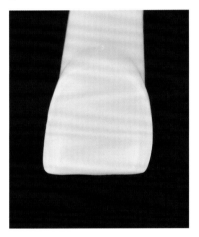

Fig 3-47　The preparation is finished on the labial view

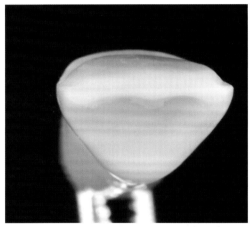

Fig 3-48　The preparation is finished on the incisal view

7. Preparation of Palatal Margin（Overlap Type）

Based on the butt-joint type veneer preparation，add the palatal overlap form to finish the preparation of the overlap type veneer. Replace it by a 1.0mm diameter round-end tapered diamond bur. On the palatal surface of the finished butt-joint type preparation incisal edge，the bur is extended for producing a 1.0mm deep and 0.5mm wide margin line，at least 1.0mm away from the contact area(Fig 3-49). The occlusal contact area or contact line locates on the healthy tissue or restoration，but should not locate on the margin line of the restoration. The palatal margin is extended to wrap the incisal edge and connects to the mesial-distal margin line naturally(Fig 3-50).

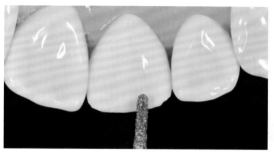

图 3-49 腭侧预备出深度 1.0mm、宽度 0.5mm 的腭侧边缘线

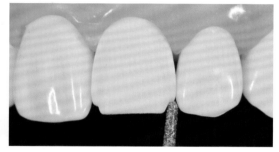

图 3-50 腭侧边缘线向近远中绕过切角与唇面近远中边缘线相延续且自然移行

八、边缘修整，精修完成（包绕型）

最后做预备体的边缘线修整、精修及磨光。使用细粒度的末端直径 1.0mm 的圆头锥状金刚砂车针，将预备体腭侧边缘、线角修整圆钝（图 3-51）。使用锐利的边缘修整器械修整腭侧边缘线，使边缘线光滑、连续（图 3-52）。使用金刚砂条抛光近中邻面边缘（图 3-53）及远中邻面边缘（图 3-54），消除飞边。

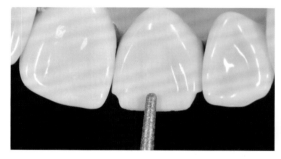

图 3-51 将预备体腭侧边缘、线角修整圆钝

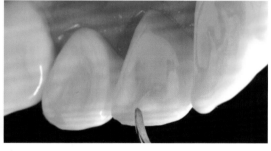

图 3-52 使用锐利的边缘修整器械修整腭侧边缘线

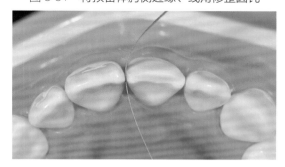

图 3-53 使用金刚砂条抛光近中邻面边缘

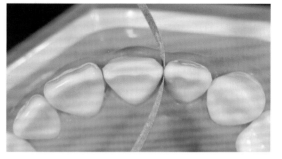

图 3-54 使用金刚砂条抛光远中邻面边缘

包绕型预备

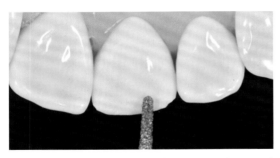

Fig 3-49　The preparation of a 1.0mm deep and 0.5mm wide palatal margin line

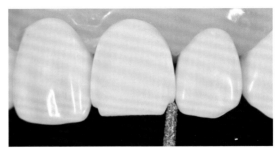

Fig 3-50　The palatal margin is extended to wrap the incisal edge and reach the mesial-distal margin line

8. Trim the Margin Line，Finish the Fine Trimming Process （Overlap Type）

Finally，trim and polish the finish line. Use a 1.0mm diameter fine-grained round-end tapered diamond to trim the marginal line of palatal surface and line angle(Fig 3-51). The sharp fringe trimmer is used to trim the margin line，which makes it smooth and continuous(Fig 3-52). Polish mesial proximal margin line(Fig 3-53) and distal proximal margin line(Fig 3-54) by dental metal polishing strips，remove the flash.

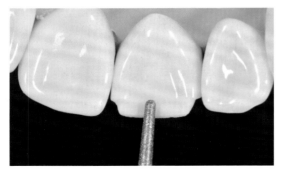

Fig 3-51　Trim the marginal line of palatal surface and line angle round

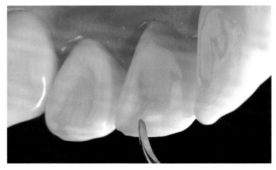

Fig 3-52　Trim the palatal margin line by sharp fringe trimmer

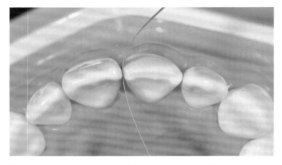

Fig 3-53　Polish mesial proximal surface margin by dental metal polishing strip

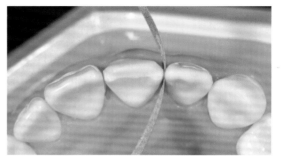

Fig 3-54　Polish distal proximal surface margin by dental metal polishing strip

九、预备体完成（包绕型）

包绕型瓷贴面牙预备体唇面观（图 3-55）、切端观（图 3-56）、腭侧面观（图 3-57）。

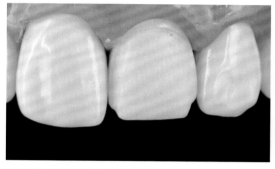 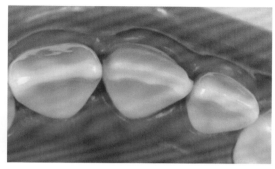

图 3-55　包绕型瓷贴面牙预备体唇面观　　　　图 3-56　包绕型瓷贴面牙预备体切端观

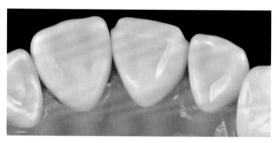

图 3-57　包绕型瓷贴面牙预备体腭侧面观

第二节　开窗型前牙瓷贴面牙体预备

开窗型前牙瓷贴面多用于牙体组织较厚、切端完整或者不需要重塑切端美观与功能情况下的贴面修复体的牙体预备。尖牙瓷贴面的牙体预备较多使用这种形式，以最大程度地保留尖牙原有的引导功能。牙体预备流程及预备量见图 3-58。

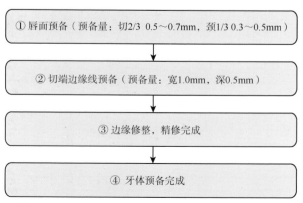

图 3-58　开窗型前牙瓷贴面牙体预备流程及预备量

9. Tooth Preparation is Finished（Overlap Type）

The labial view(Fig 3-55), the incisal view(Fig 3-56) and the palatal view(Fig 3-57) of the overlap type porcelain veneer preparation.

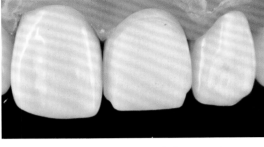

Fig 3-55　The labial view of the overlap type porcelain veneer preparation

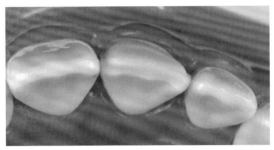

Fig 3-56　The incisal view of the overlap type porcelain veneer preparation

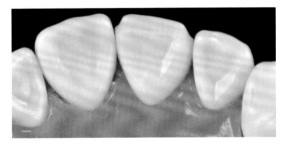

Fig 3-57　The palatal view of the overlap type porcelain veneer preparation

Section 2　Window Type Porcelain Veneer Preparation of Anterior Tooth

The window type veneer adapts to the conditions including that: the tissue is thick, the incisal edge is intact and does not reshape the contour and recover the function. It is widely used in canine tooth to keep the original guidance function. The preparation of canine tooth process and reduction are shown in Fig 3-58.

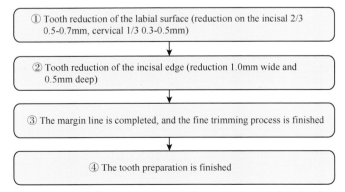

① Tooth reduction of the labial surface (reduction on the incisal 2/3 0.5-0.7mm, cervical 1/3 0.3-0.5mm)

② Tooth reduction of the incisal edge (reduction 1.0mm wide and 0.5mm deep)

③ The margin line is completed, and the fine trimming process is finished

④ The tooth preparation is finished

Fig 3-58　Window type porcelain veneer preparation process and reduction of anterior tooth

一、唇面预备

下文以 23 牙为例介绍开窗型瓷贴面的牙体预备。首先是唇面预备，分为两步：①唇面深度指示沟预备；②唇面牙体组织磨除。

第一步：唇面深度指示沟的预备。上颌尖牙的外形高点线多位于切 2/3 与颈 1/3 的交界处，上前牙唇面的牙釉质量从切端到颈部是逐步减少的，并且切 2/3 对美学效果要求更高，唇面的预备量从切 2/3 的 0.5 ～ 0.7mm 到颈 1/3 的 0.3 ～ 0.5mm 逐步减少，所以唇面需分别在切 2/3 和颈 1/3 制备 0.5mm 和 0.3mm 的深度指示沟。

使用刃深 0.5mm 的深度指示车针，在唇面切 1/3 处和中 1/3 处制备两条约 0.5mm 的深度指示沟，刃部完全没入（图 3-59）。车针放置方向：车针柄与切 2/3 轴面平行一致（图 3-60），使用车针柄的光滑部分防止切入过深，此时切勿将车针柄翘起脱离牙齿轴面。

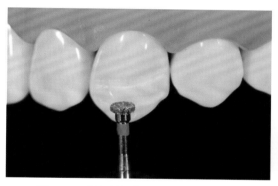

图 3-59　制备唇面切 2/3 的深度指示沟

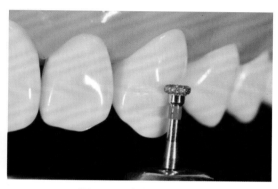

图 3-60　车针放置方向

切 2/3 轴面 0.5mm 的深度指示沟制备完成，唇面观（图 3-61），此时在深度指示沟底涂上颜色标记，近中面观（图 3-62），指示沟走行与原牙近远中斜面一致。

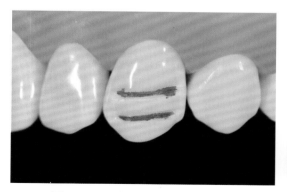

图 3-61　深度指示沟完成，唇面观

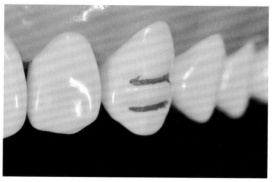

图 3-62　深度指示沟完成，近中面观

1. Preparation of Labial Surface

The following takes 23 teeth as an example to introduce the preparation process of the window type porcelain veneer. The first step is the labial surface preparation, which is divided into two stages: the preparation of labial surface depth grooves and the removement of the tissue between the grooves.

First step is the preparation of labial surface depth grooves. The height line of contour locates in the junction between the incisal 2/3 and cervical 1/3 of the labial surface. In view of the gradual decrease amount of the enamel from incisal to cervical part and more demand esthetics achieved in incisal 2/3 labial surface, so the reduction is 0.3-0.5mm on cervical 1/3 decreasing from the 0.5-0.7mm of the incisal 2/3. 0.5mm deep depth orientation grooves on incisal 2/3, and 0.3mm deep on cervical 1/3 are prepared respectively.

Use the depth-marker bur with 0.5mm-deep blade to make two 0.5mm deep depth orientation grooves on incisal 1/3 and middle 1/3 of the labial surface respectively. The blade is sunk into the tooth(Fig 3-59). The direction of the bur: the bur parallels the incisal 2/3 axial surface (Fig 3-60). The smooth part of the bur stem is used to prevent cutting too much tissue, do not detach the bur stem from the tooth.

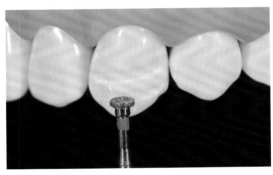 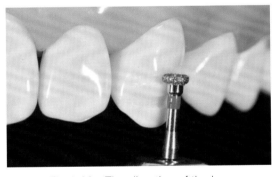

Fig 3-59 Preparation of depth grooves on incisal 2/3 of labial surface

Fig 3-60 The direction of the bur

The preparation of 0.5mm depth grooves of incisal 2/3 axial surface is finished on the labial view(Fig 3-61). Color the bottom of the depth grooves as marks. On the mesial view, the grooves follow the mesiodistal slope of the uncut tooth(Fig 3-62).

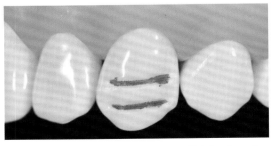 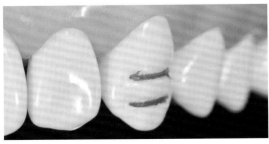

Fig 3-61 The depth grooves are finished on the labial view

Fig 3-62 The depth grooves are finished on the mesial view

　　切 2/3 深度指示沟预备完成后，换用刃深 0.3mm 的深度指示车针，在唇面颈 1/3 制备一条深约 0.3mm 的深度指示沟（图 3-63），刃部完全没入。车针放置方向：车针柄与颈 1/3 轴面平行（图 3-64），同样车针柄切勿脱离颈 1/3 轴面，防止切入过深。

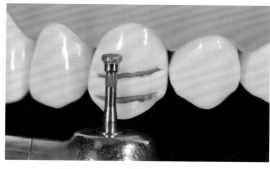 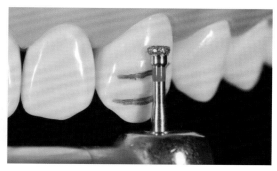

图 3-63　唇面制备深度指示沟　　　　　　　图 3-64　车针放置方向

　　唇面深度指示沟预备完成（图 3-65），在指示沟底标记上颜色。
　　第二步：深度指示沟间牙体组织磨除，仍然按照切 2/3 及颈 1/3 两个轴面来预备。更换末端直径 1.0mm 的圆头锥状金刚砂车针，车针沿与唇面切 2/3 轴面平行的方向，按照深度指示沟指示的深度，磨除切 2/3 远中到近中边缘嵴之间的牙体组织（图 3-66）。同时在近远中边缘嵴处，向邻接区扩展，最大可进入邻接区的一半，但不破坏接触点，形成近远中邻面内线角圆钝的边缘线，防止在侧向观时边缘线暴露出来，预备时应避免伤及邻牙。近中面观车针放置方向：车针柄与 2/3 轴面平行接触，边缘线位于邻接区内（图 3-67）。
　　完成唇面切 2/3 牙体组织磨除（图 3-68）。

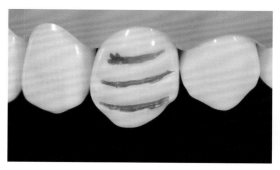 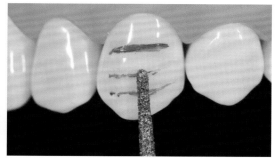

图 3-65　唇面深度指示沟完成　　　　　　　图 3-66　磨除切 2/3 牙体组织

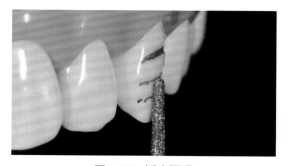 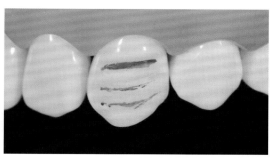

图 3-67　近中面观　　　　　　　　　　　　图 3-68　切 2/3 牙体组织磨除完成

After the preparation of depth grooves on incisal 2/3 labial surface is finished, use a depth-marker bur with 0.3mm deep blade to make an approximately 0.3mm depth groove on cervical 1/3 labial surface(Fig 3-63). The blade is sunk into the tissue completely. The direction of the bur: the bur stem is parallel to the cervical 1/3 axial surface(Fig 3-64). Do not detach the bur stem from the tooth in case of cutting too much tissue.

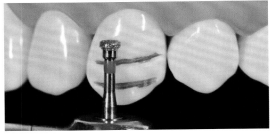 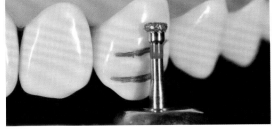

Fig 3-63 Preparation of the labial depth grooves   Fig 3-64 The direction of the bur

The preparation of depth grooves on the labial surface is finished(Fig 3-65). Color the bottom of the grooves as marks.

Next, remove the tissue between the depth orientation grooves. The step is still separated by the incisal 2/3 and cervical 1/3 part respectively. A 1.0mm diameter round-end tapered diamond is replaced. The bur is parallel to the incisal 2/3 labial surface to remove the tissue from the distal to mesial marginal ridges on incisal 2/3 surface(Fig 3-66). The bur is extended up to half of the proximal surface without damage to the contact area on the mesial and distal marginal ridge, which forms the round marginal line, in case of exposing the finish line on the proximal view. Take care not to damage the adjacent tooth. The direction of the bur on the mesial view: the bur contacts the 2/3 axial surface parallelly, the margin line locates in the contact area(Fig 3-67).

The removing of the incisal 2/3 of labial surface is finished(Fig 3-68).

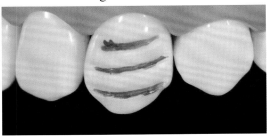 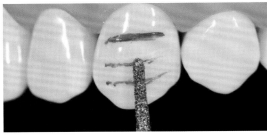

Fig 3-65 The preparation of depth orientation   Fig 3-66 The removing tissue on incisal 2/3 labial
grooves on labial surface is finished   surface

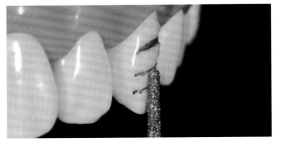 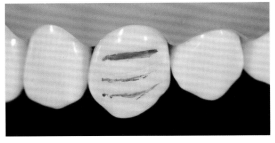

Fig 3-67 The mesial view   Fig 3-68 The removing of the incisal 2/3 labial
surface is finished

然后是颈 1/3 深度指示沟间的牙体组织磨除，使用同一车针沿与唇面颈 1/3 轴面平行的方向，按照深度指示沟指示的深度，磨除颈 1/3 远中到近中边缘嵴之间的牙体组织（图 3-69）。在颈部预备至平齐龈缘处，形成 0.3 ～ 0.4mm 宽、内线角圆钝的颈部边缘线。

在近远中边缘嵴处，向非自洁区扩展，形成近远中龈外展隙处边缘线，与切 2/3 边缘线及颈部边缘线分别延续（图 3-70），预备时避免伤及邻牙。

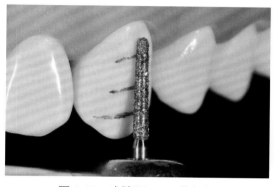

图 3-69　磨除颈 1/3 牙体组织

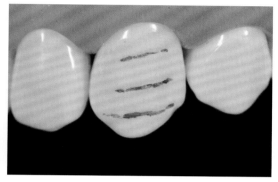

图 3-70　边缘线移行过渡

完成唇面预备，近中面观（图 3-71），近远中邻面边缘线均位于非自洁区，唇面预备完成时，深度指示沟底的颜色标记线不能完全被磨除，这样可以有效防止预备过量。

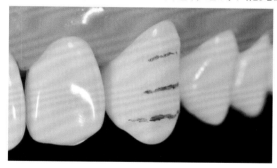

图 3-71　近中面观

开窗型唇面预备

二、切端边缘线预备

开窗型瓷贴面的牙体预备在第一步时基本上与对接型瓷贴面牙体预备方法一致，但这种预备形式与对接型预备最大的不同就是其需在患牙切端的唇面再预备出一条宽 1.0mm、深 0.5mm 的边缘线，并与近远中邻面边缘线自然延续贯通，这对患牙切端的厚度就提出了一定的要求。

使用末端直径 1.0mm 的圆头锥状金刚砂车针在切端顺应牙尖走行制备出宽度 1mm、深度 0.5mm 的切端边缘线（图 3-72）。

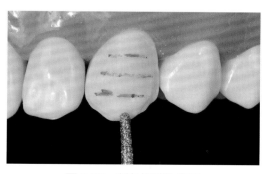

图 3-72　制备切端边缘线

Then，the tissue between the depth orientation grooves on cervical 1/3 is removed. The same bur is parallel to the cervical 1/3 labial surface. The tissue from distal to mesial marginal ridges on cervical 1/3 surface is removed according to the depth of the grooves(Fig 3-69). The cervical finish line is ended at the gingival margin and of uniform 0.3-0.4mm width with a round internal line angle.

Extend the bur to the non-self-cleaning area on the distal marginal ridge，which forms margin line in the mesiodistal gingival embrasure. The margin line connects to the incisal 2/3 and cervical marginal line(Fig 3-70). Take care not to damage the adjacent tooth.

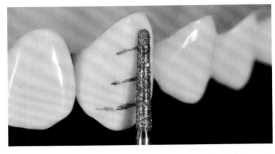 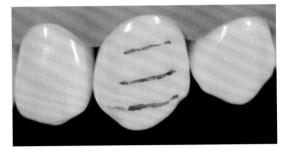

Fig 3-69　Removing the tissue on cervical 1/3 part　　Fig 3-70　The finish lines transit naturally

On the mesial view，the labial surface preparation is finished(Fig 3-71). The margin lines of the mesiodistal proximal surface locate in non-self-cleaning area. When the preparation is finished，the depth groove marker is not totally removed to avoid the over-preparation.

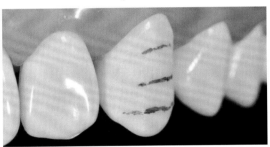

Fig 3-71　The mesial view

2. Preparation of Margin Line on Incisal Edge

The first step of window type preparation is the same as the butt-joint type veneer preparation.

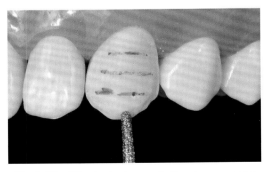

Fig 3-72　The incisal margin line is prepared

However，there is a big difference between this two type preparation：the window type veneer preparation needs to make a 1.0mm wide，0.5mm deep finish line on the labial surface connected with the proximal surface marginal line naturally，which makes the request for the incisal edge thickness.

Use a 1.0mm diameter round-end tapered diamond bur following the contour of the uncut cusp on the incisal edge to make a 1.0mm wide，0.5mm deep finish margin on incisal edge(Fig 3-72).

预备后的唇面观切端边缘线完全顺应牙尖走行（图 3-73），近中面观（图 3-74）。

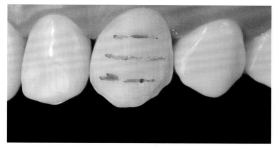
图 3-73　唇面观

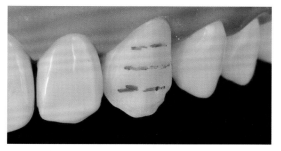
图 3-74　近中面观

开窗型边缘线预备

三、边缘修整，精修完成

完成上述步骤后，开窗型贴面的牙体初预备完成，然后是预备体的边缘修整及精修与磨光。换用细粒度末端直径为 1.0mm 的圆头锥状金刚砂车针，分别将预备体近远中颈部边缘及切端边缘线修整圆钝光滑（图 3-75～图 3-77），边缘线宽 0.3～0.5mm，内线角圆钝，边缘线沿上颌尖牙的解剖外形自然延续，形成 360° 的环状结构。

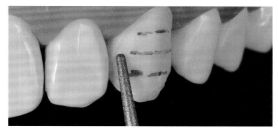
图 3-75　近远中边缘线修整

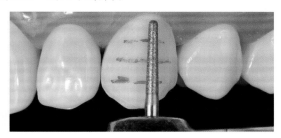
图 3-76　颈部边缘线修整

使用同一车针适度磨光唇面牙体组织（图 3-78），并使所有的线角、面角、轴角圆钝光滑。此时唇面的颜色标记线完全消除，达到设计的预备量。

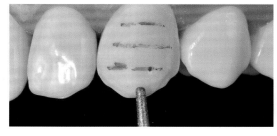
图 3-77　切端边缘线修整

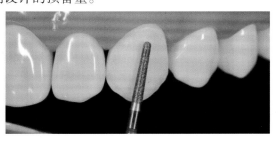
图 3-78　磨光唇面牙体组织

The marginal line follows the cusp completely on the labial view(Fig 3-73). The mesial view(Fig 3-74).

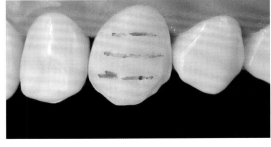

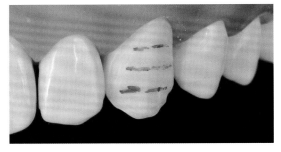

Fig 3-73　The labial view

Fig 3-74　The mesial view

3. Margin Line is Prepared，and Fine Trimming Process is Finished

The initial preparation of the window type veneer is finished after the mentioned steps above. Then the marginal line needs to be trimmed，fine trimmed and polished. The bur is replaced by a 1.0mm diameter fine-grained round-end tapered diamond. The finish line of mesiodistal cervical part and incisal edge is trimmed to round and smooth(Fig 3-75-Fig 3-77). The finish line is 0.3-0.5mm wide with a round internal line angle. The marginal line forms a 360° cyclic structure moving naturally along the anatomical contour of the canine tooth.

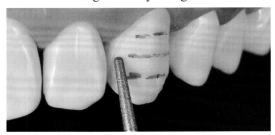

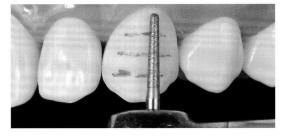

Fig 3-75　The mesial and distal finish lines are trimmed

Fig 3-76　The trimming process of the cervical margin

Polish the labial tissue moderately by the fine-grained bur(Fig 3-78) and make all line angles，plane angles and axial angles round and smooth. The depth groove markers are removed totally to acquire the reduction.

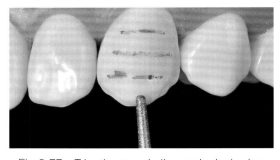

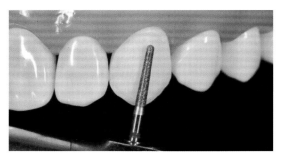

Fig 3-77　Trim the margin line on incisal edge

Fig 3-78　Polish the labial surface

为了获得更加清晰、准确的边缘线，从而有更加理想的修复体边缘适合性，使用锐利的边缘修整器械修整所有的边缘线（图 3-79），使边缘线光滑、连续。

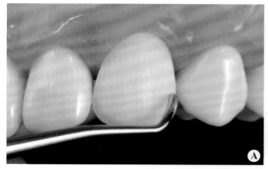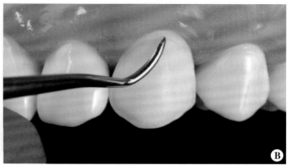

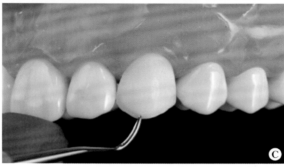

图 3-79　修整近远中边缘线（Ａ），唇面颈部边缘线（Ｂ），切端边缘线（Ｃ）

对于车针及锐利边缘修整器械不易到达的近中及远中邻面接触区，使用金刚砂条抛光近中邻面边缘（图 3-80）及远中邻面边缘（图 3-81），使预备体与邻牙轻度分离，也方便获得清晰的印模及可卸石膏代型。

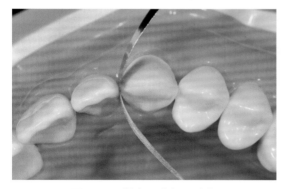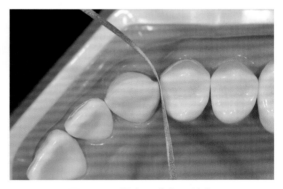

图 3-80　抛光近中邻面边缘　　　　　图 3-81　抛光远中邻面边缘

开窗型精修与磨光

73

To acquire a margin line more clear and accurate, get the restoration margin more dense to the preparation, the sharp fringe trimmer is used to trim the marginal line(Fig 3-79), which blends the finish line smooth and continuous.

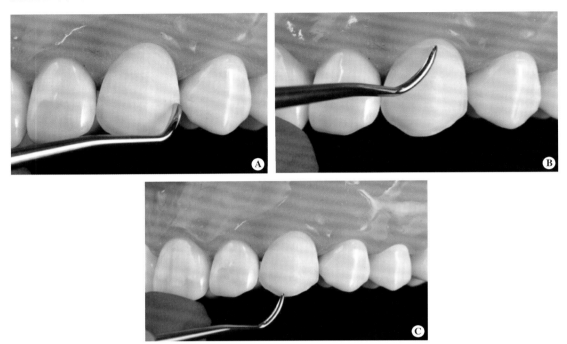

Fig 3-79   The trimming process of the mesial and distal margins（A）, the cervical margins（B）, the incisal margins（C）

The mesiodistal proximal contact area is too difficult for the trimmer to get through, so we use metal polishing strip to polish the mesial proximal surface margin(Fig 3-80) and distal proximal surface margin(Fig 3-81) to separate it from the adjacent tooth slightly. In this way, the impression would be clear and the generation easy to be moved.

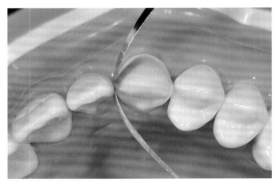

Fig 3-80   Polish mesial proximal surface margin

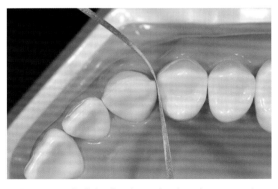

Fig 3-81   Polish distal proximal surface margin

四、预备体完成

开窗型瓷贴面牙体预备完成唇面观（图 3-82），仍保留了预备原牙的解剖轮廓外形。牙体预备完成近中面观（图 3-83），邻面边缘线均位于不易暴露的非自洁区。

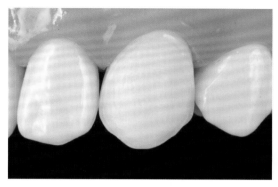

图 3-82　唇面观

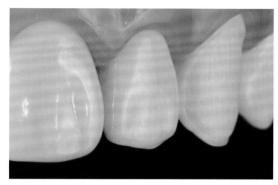

图 3-83　近中面观

完成的预备体（图 3-84A），黄色标线是 360° 边缘线（图 3-84B）。

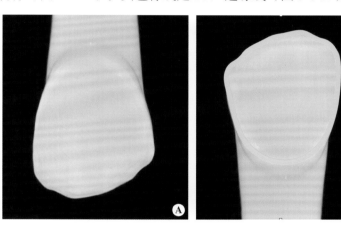

图 3-84　完成的预备体

4. Tooth Preparation is Finished

The labial view after the preparation of window type porcelain veneer(Fig 3-82), which keeps the anatomical contour of the uncut tooth.

The mesial view after the preparation(Fig 3-83), the proximal marginal line locates in invisible non-self-cleaning area.

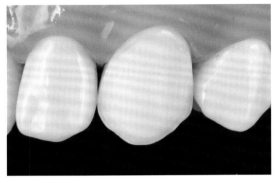
Fig 3-82   The labial view

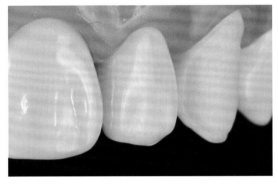
Fig 3-83   The mesial view

The finished preparation(Fig 3-84A). The yellow line is a 360° margin line(Fig 3-84B).

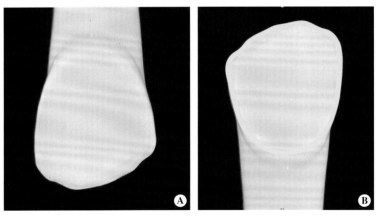
Fig 3-84   The finished preparation

第四章　磨牙嵌体预备

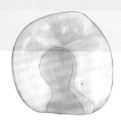

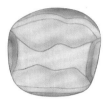

近年来，嵌体（inlay）以其较好的美学性能受到越来越多口腔医生的重视及患者的青睐。但是嵌体有着自身的特点，如拉应力特点，因此在临床应用时要比全冠更加小心，临床上嵌体预备并没有完全一致的模式，这一点与全冠不同，嵌体预备多会按照牙体缺损的情况来设计，形式多种多样。

嵌体是一种嵌入牙体组织内部，用以恢复牙体缺损患牙形态和功能的修复体。嵌体采用冠内固位体，由缺损患牙剩余的牙体组织所包绕，固位方式主要是洞固位形。嵌体受力时将应力传导至固位形的侧壁后在剩余牙体内部产生拉应力，而牙釉质、牙本质的力学特征是抗压而不抗拉，过大的拉应力会造成牙体折裂，所以嵌体是一种能修复牙体组织缺损而不能为剩余牙体组织提供保护的修复体。采用嵌体修复时要求剩余牙体组织有足够强度来提供抗力并保证修复体的固位，一般用于修复牙体缺损量较小的患牙。这一特点应作为考虑是否使用嵌体修复的首要因素。

嵌体有很多种，根据嵌体覆盖牙面的不同，可以分为单面嵌体、双面嵌体和多面嵌体，本章以下颌磨牙邻𬌗面双面嵌体及高嵌体制备为例进行牙体预备示教，预备流程及预备量见图 4-1。

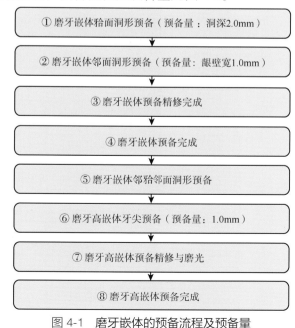

① 磨牙嵌体𬌗面洞形预备（预备量：洞深2.0mm）

② 磨牙嵌体邻面洞形预备（预备量：龈壁宽1.0mm）

③ 磨牙嵌体预备精修完成

④ 磨牙嵌体预备完成

⑤ 磨牙嵌体邻𬌗邻面洞形预备

⑥ 磨牙高嵌体牙尖预备（预备量：1.0mm）

⑦ 磨牙高嵌体预备精修与磨光

⑧ 磨牙高嵌体预备完成

图 4-1　磨牙嵌体的预备流程及预备量

Chapter 4　Inlay Preparation of Molar Tooth

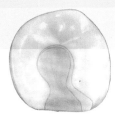

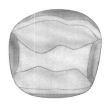

In recent years, the inlay gets increasing attention from the dentists because of the excellent esthetics, and it is popular among the patients. However, there are several unique features of this restoration, such as the tension force, which demands more careful clinic application. The process of preparation is not consistent, which is different from the all-crown. The designation adapts to the defect variously.

The inlay is fabricated as to fit into the inner part of the tooth. The inlay is made precisely to restore the shape and function of the defect tooth. The inlay adapts the intracoronal retainer, surrounded by the remaining tissue of the defected tooth, the main retention form of which is hole shape retention. When the inlay is stressed, the force is transmitted to the side wall of the cavity to produce the tensile force inside the remaining tooth. However, the mechanical characteristics of enamel and dentin can resist the pressure not the tensile.

Excessive tensile stress will cause tooth fracture. Therefore, the inlay is a restoration that can repair the defect of the tooth, but it cannot provide protection for the remaining tooth structure. When using inlays for restoration, the tooth must have sufficient structure to resist fracture and ensure the success of restoration. Usually inlays are used to repair minor tooth structure defects, which should be primary factor to consider whether we choose this kind of restoration.

There are many types of inlay. According to the different covered tooth surfaces, they can be categorized into single-sided inlay, double-sided inlay and multi-sided inlay. This chapter shows the procedure of proximal occlusal. D double-sided inlay and onlay preparation on the lower molar tooth. The preparation process and reduction is shown in Fig 4-1.

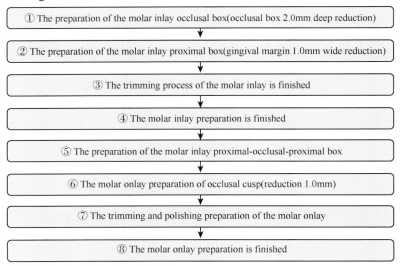

① The preparation of the molar inlay occlusal box(occlusal box 2.0mm deep reduction)

↓

② The preparation of the molar inlay proximal box(gingival margin 1.0mm wide reduction)

↓

③ The trimming process of the molar inlay is finished

↓

④ The molar inlay preparation is finished

↓

⑤ The preparation of the molar inlay proximal-occlusal-proximal box

↓

⑥ The molar onlay preparation of occlusal cusp(reduction 1.0mm)

↓

⑦ The trimming and polishing preparation of the molar onlay

↓

⑧ The molar onlay preparation is finished

Fig 4-1　Inlay preparation process and reduction of molar tooth

第一节　磨牙邻𬌗嵌体牙体预备

一、𬌗面洞形预备

嵌体能够在口内发挥作用的前提是它能牢固地与患牙连在一起，其固位力主要来自于机械固位，辅以粘接固位，机械固位又主要依赖于洞固位形及鸠尾固位。嵌体预备首先从𬌗面洞形预备开始。

使用小球形金刚砂车针，去除𬌗面洞内腐质（图4-2），蓝色标记是龋坏牙体组织，同时去除洞壁周围薄弱的牙体组织并消除洞内倒凹（图4-3）。

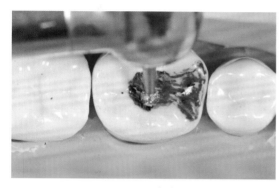

图 4-2　去腐

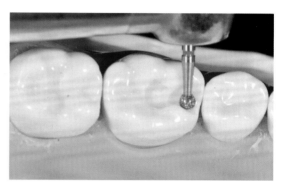

图 4-3　去除薄壁弱尖

然后换用平头圆角短粗状金刚砂车针，沿着去腐洞形制备𬌗面洞形（图4-4），洞深为2.0mm，洞底平直或浅凹形，内线角圆钝，各轴壁𬌗向外展约6°，与嵌体就位道方向一致，𬌗面洞形边缘需避开咬合接触区至少1.0mm。

𬌗面洞形制备完成（图4-5），洞深为2.0mm，洞底平或浅凹形，内线角圆钝。颊舌轴壁𬌗向外展合计约12°，方便嵌体的顺利就位。

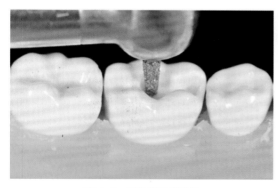

图 4-4　𬌗面洞形制备

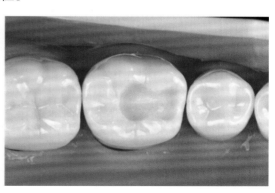

图 4-5　𬌗面洞形制备完成

Section 1 Proximal-Occlusal Inlay Preparation of Molar Tooth

1. Preparation of Occlusal Cavity

The inlay function in oral under the condition that it connects to the tooth closely. The retention derives mainly from mechanical retention assisted by attachment. The former depends on the cavity retainer and the dovetail retainer. The first step is to prepare the occlusal cavity.

The small round diamond bur is used to remove all carious lesions on occlusal cavity (Fig 4-2). The blue mark is the decayed tissue. Remove all weak tissue around the walls and the undercut(Fig 4-3).

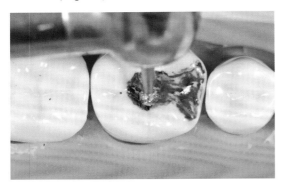
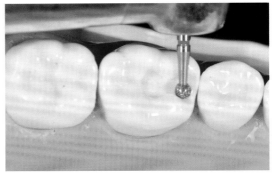

Fig 4-2　Remove all carious lesions　　Fig 4-3　Remove all thin walls and unsupported cusps

A flat-end cylindrical diamond replaced the bur to prepare the occlusal cavity along the decay outline(Fig 4-4). The cavity is 2.0mm deep. The bottom of the cavity is flat or concave slightly. The internal line angles are round. All axial walls are about 6° divergence，which is consistent to the path of insertion of the inlay. The depth of the occlusal outline ends at least 1.0mm from the occlusal contact area.

The occlusal outline is finished(Fig 4-5). The depth is 2.0mm. The cavity bottom is flat or concave slightly. The internal line angles are round. The buccal and lingual axial walls are about 12° divergence，which is convenient for inlay to insert.

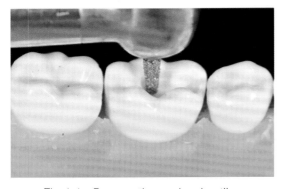
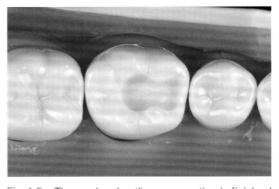

Fig 4-4　Prepare the occlusal outline　　Fig 4-5　The occlusal outline preparation is finished

去净腐质及𬌗面薄弱牙体组织后，将𬌗面洞形向近中邻面边缘嵴扩展（图 4-6），包括邻近的点隙、发育沟等，使洞缘线均位于自洁区的健康牙体组织。

𬌗面洞形完成时，需沿着牙尖形态制备出鸠尾固位形（图 4-7），防止嵌体近远中向脱位。鸠尾设计一般遵循以下原则：峡部放在两个相对牙尖三角嵴之间，宽度为颊舌尖宽度的 1/3 ～ 1/2，或宽度至少为 2.0mm。

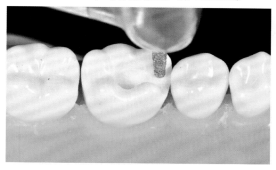

图 4-6　𬌗面洞形向近中邻面边缘嵴扩展

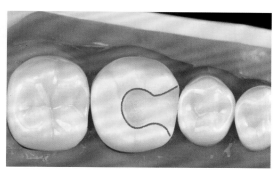

图 4-7　制备出鸠尾固位形

𬌗面洞形预备

二、邻面洞形预备

在𬌗面完成 2.0mm 洞深及鸠尾状洞形预备后，开始进入近中邻面箱状洞形的预备，换用直径为 1.0mm 的圆角柱状金刚砂车针向邻面根方制备邻面箱状洞形（图 4-8），并向外扩展颊舌轴壁，使其边缘线均位于颊舌侧外展隙的自洁区。颊舌轴壁外展约 12°，与嵌体𬌗面就位道方向保持一致。龈壁向根方预备至自洁区，形成内线角圆钝的龈壁边缘线，宽约 1.0mm。预备后龈壁及颊舌轴壁均为平直状态，龈壁应与邻牙分离。

如果邻接区较大，龈壁不易与邻牙分离时使用细针状金刚砂车针深入邻接区，轻轻打开邻接（图 4-9），做到与邻牙分离。预备时车针尽量向患牙方向用力，切勿伤及邻牙。

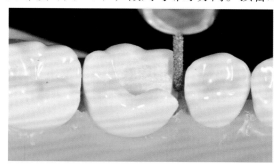

图 4-8　制备邻面箱状洞形

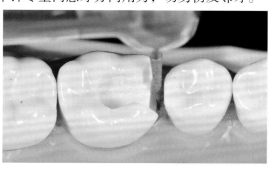

图 4-9　打开邻接

When the decayed tissue and weak tooth are removed, the occlusal outline is extended to mesial proximal marginal ridge(Fig 4-6), which includes the adjacent grooves and pits. The box margin is located at the self-cleaning area of the healthy tissue.

When the occlusal box preparation is finished, the occlusal dovetail is added along the cusp contour(Fig 4-7). For preventing dislocating mesiodistally, the design of the dovetail should follow these principles: the dovetail form isthmus lays on the middle of the opposite cusps, triangular ridges, the width of which is 1/3-1/2 of the distance between the buccal and lingual cusps, at least 2.0mm wide.

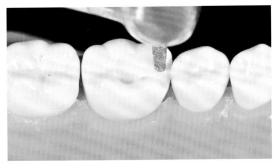

Fig 4-6　The occlusal outline is extended to proximal marginal ridge

Fig 4-7　Prepare the dovetail retentive form

2. Preparation of Proximal Box

Prepare the proximal box after the preparation of 2.0mm deep occlusal cavity and dovetail form cavity. Replace the bur by a round-end tapered diamond with a diameter of 1.0mm to produce the proximal box towards the root(Fig 4-8). The axial walls are extended facially and lingually into the self-cleaning area. All axial walls are smooth and about 12° divergence, which is consistent with the path of insertion of the inlay. The root of the gingival wall is prepared to self-cleaning area, to form the shoulder with the internal line angles, the width of the gingival wall is about 1.0mm. The gingival wall and axial wall should keep straight, and the gingival wall should be separated from the adjacent tooth after the preparation.

If the contact area is too broad to open, the gingival wall is difficult to separate from the adjacent tooth, the sharp-tipped flame diamond is used to enter the contact area, cut the curving proximal surface of the tooth slightly until the contact is opened(Fig 4-9). Force the bur towards the prepared tooth without damage to the adjacent tooth.

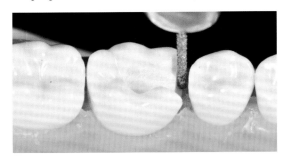
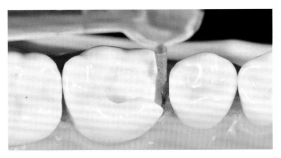

Fig 4-8　Preparation of the proximal box

Fig 4-9　Opening the contact

　　完成的邻面洞形，颊舌轴壁外展约 12°，与嵌体𬌗面就位道方向一致。龈壁及颊舌轴壁均预备至自洁区，内线角圆钝。

　　颊面观（图 4-10），𬌗面观（图 4-11）。

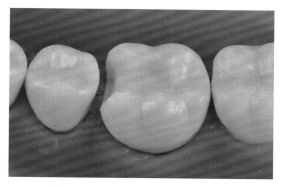
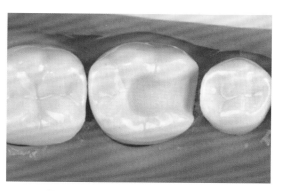

图 4-10　完成的邻面洞形：颊面观　　　　图 4-11　完成的邻面洞形：𬌗面观

邻面洞形预备

三、精 修 完 成

　　𬌗面及邻面洞形预备完成后剩余颊舌壁厚度均应不小于 2.0mm，否则不能很好地抵抗嵌体戴入后给剩余牙体组织带来的拉应力，尤其是邻面洞的颊舌轴壁须能抵抗足够大的拉应力，才能保证嵌体长期使用，防止剩余牙体组织折裂。

　　下一步是对预备体进行精修与磨光，使用细粒度的平头圆角状金刚砂车针将预备体𬌗面洞（图 4-12）及邻面洞（图 4-13）轴壁、各边缘、内线角修整圆钝，磨光预备体。

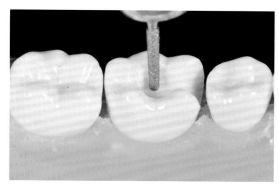
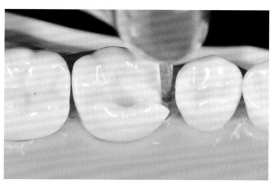

图 4-12　𬌗面洞形磨光　　　　　　　　图 4-13　邻面洞形磨光

The finished proximal box. All axial walls are about 12° divergence, which is consistent with the path of insertion of the inlay. The gingival wall and axial wall are prepared to self-cleaning area. The internal corner is round.

The buccal view (Fig 4-10) and the occlusal view (Fig 4-11).

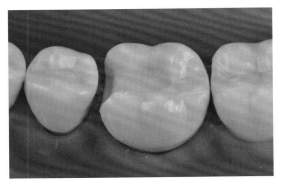

Fig 4-10　The buccal view of the finished proximal box

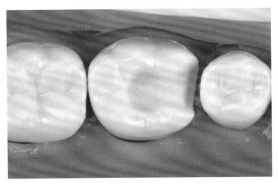

Fig 4-11　The occlusal view of the finished proximal box

3. Fine Trimming Process is Finished

The thickness of buccal and lingual wall is at least 2.0mm to bear the tension force to the remaining tissue when the onlay/inlay is put into the oral cavity, especially the buccal and lingual wall of the proximal cavity must resist the enough tension for long-standing use, in case that the remaining tissue breaks off.

Next is to trim and polish. Replace the bur by the flat-end finishing bur with round-angle, trim the occlusal cavity(Fig 4-12) and proximal cavity(Fig 4-13) axial walls, margin and internal line angles. Polish the preparation.

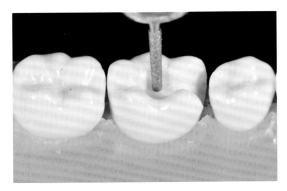

Fig 4-12　The occlusal box is polished

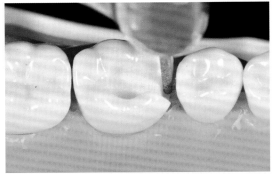

Fig 4-13　The proximal box is polished

　　最后使用锐利的边缘修整器械修整龈壁边缘线（图4-14），使边缘线光滑、连续，消除飞边。

　　完成的预备体𬌗面观（图4-15）。𬌗面呈鸠尾洞形，邻面呈倒梯形，以利于嵌体就位。

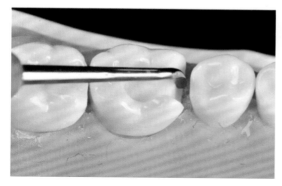

图4-14　龈壁边缘线修整

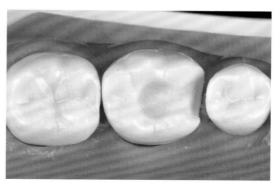

图4-15　完成的预备体𬌗面观

四、预备体完成

　　牙体预备完成𬌗面观（图4-16），洞形底平壁直，内线角圆钝，红色标线为𬌗面鸠尾形洞缘线。

　　牙体预备完成近中邻面观（图4-17），邻面洞形颊舌轴壁（红色标线）分别与𬌗面洞形颊舌轴壁（黄色标线）平行，邻面洞边缘线（红色标线）位于自洁区。

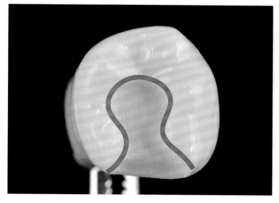

图4-16　牙体预备完成𬌗面观

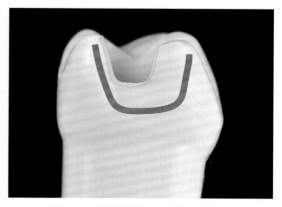

图4-17　牙体预备完成近中邻面观

At last the sharp fringe trimmer is used to trim the margin line of gingival wall(Fig 4-14), which blends the margin line smooth and continuous. Remove the flash.

The occlusal view of the finished preparation(Fig 4-15). The occlusal surface shows the dovetail cavity，and the proximal surface shows inverted trapezoidal，which is available for inlay to insert to the tooth.

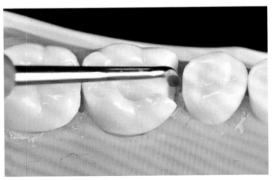
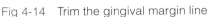

Fig 4-14　Trim the gingival margin line

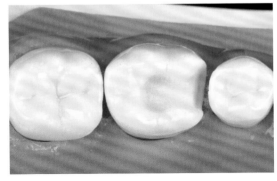

Fig 4-15　The occlusal view of tooth preparation

4. Tooth Preparation is Finished

The finished preparation on the occlusal view(Fig 4-16). The pulpal floor is flat and the axial wall is straight. The internal line angles are round. Red line is the outline of occlusal dovetail.

The finished preparation on the proximal view(Fig 4-17). The buccal and lingual walls of the proximal box(red line) are parallel to those of the occlusal box(yellow line). The proximal box marginal line(red line) is located at the self-cleaning area.

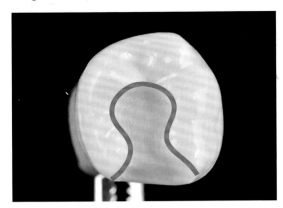

Fig 4-16　The occlusal view after preparation

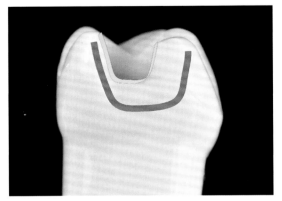

Fig 4-17　The mesial proximal view after preparation

第二节　磨牙高嵌体牙体预备

高嵌体是指覆盖了部分或者全部牙尖的嵌体特殊形式，既有嵌入牙体组织的部分，又有包绕覆盖牙尖，甚至包绕部分轴面的情况。在完成邻𬌗洞形的制备后，再增加牙尖的预备即可完成高嵌体牙体预备。

一、邻𬌗邻面洞形预备

首先将磨牙近中邻𬌗面洞形增加预备成邻𬌗邻面洞形。

按照本章第一节磨牙邻𬌗嵌体预备的方法，分别在𬌗面远中部分及远中邻面预备远中邻𬌗面嵌体洞形，𬌗面洞在中部近远中向贯通（图4-18），𬌗面洞缘线呈双鸠尾形状（图4-19），红色标记的边缘线均位于自洁区且避开咬合接触区至少1.0mm，洞形内底平壁直，内线角圆钝。

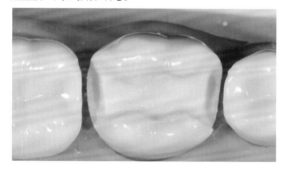

图4-18　邻𬌗邻面洞形预备

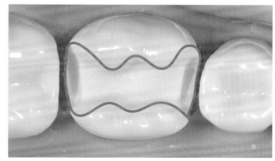

图4-19　𬌗面双鸠尾固位形

高嵌体邻𬌗邻面洞形预备

二、牙尖预备

下面是牙尖预备，即预备修复体覆盖牙尖的空间，分为功能尖和非功能尖预备。

功能尖预备包括颊斜面、舌斜面两部分。首先是功能尖颊斜面深度指示沟预备，使用直径1.0mm圆角柱状金刚砂车针在下颌后牙功能尖颊斜面预备4～5条深度为1.0mm的指示沟（图4-20），恰好为没入一根车针的量，建议将指示沟分别定在牙尖嵴顶及牙尖窝沟底。

预备完成的下颌后牙功能尖颊斜面深度指示沟（图4-21）。

Section 2　Tooth Preparation of Molar Onlay

The onlay is a type of restoration that covers part of or a whole cusp, the preparation process contains inserting into the tooth, covering the cusp and even wrapping around the part of the axial surface. After the preparation of the proximal-occlusal cavity, preparing the cusp additionally can finish the onlay preparation.

1. Preparation of Proximal-Occlusal-Proximal Cavity

Firstly, prepare the mesioocclusal cavity to proximal-occlusal-proximal cavity.

According to the preparation of molar proximal-occlusal inlay describing in part one of this chapter, prepare the proximal-occlusal onlay cavity on distal occlusal surface and distal proximal surface. Connect the mesial and distal reduction on the center of occlusal cavity (Fig 4-18). The occlusal outline presents a double dovetail form(Fig 4-19). The red marker locates in self- cleaning area and avoids touching the occlusal contact area at least 1.0mm. The pulpal floor is flat and the axial wall is straight.

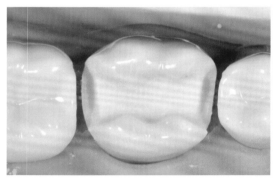 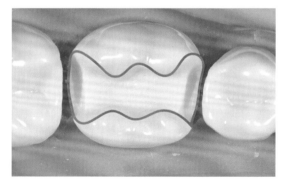

Fig 4-18　The preparation of proximal-occlusal-proximal cavity

Fig 4-19　The occlusal view of the double dovetail retentive form

2. Preparation of Cusp

The next is to prepare the cusps to fabricate the space for the restoration covering the cusp, which includes functional cusp and nonfunctional cusp.

The preparation of functional cusp contains the buccal bevel and the lingual bevel. The first thing is the preparation of the depth grooves on buccal slope of functional cusp. Use a 1.0mm diameter round-end tapered diamond bur along the buccal inclination of the functional cusps to make 4-5 depth grooves(Fig 4-20). Making sure the diamond is inserted into the tooth to its full diameter. We recommend to locate the depth grooves on the top of the cusp ridge and the bottom of the cusp pit and fissure.

The finished depth grooves on the buccal inclination of the mandibular posterior tooth functional cusps(Fig 4-21).

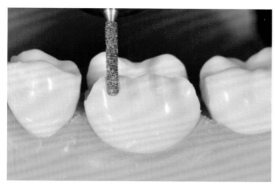

图 4-20 下颌后牙功能尖颊斜面深度指示沟预备

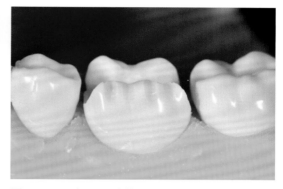

图 4-21 下颌后牙功能尖颊斜面深度指示沟预备完成

使用同一车针按照与上一步骤相同的方法在功能尖舌斜面预备 3 ～ 4 条深度为 1.0mm 的指示沟（图 4-22），恰好为没入一根车针的量。

在完成功能尖颊舌斜面深度指示沟后，使用相同车针先沿功能尖颊斜面牙尖起伏走行，均匀磨除深度指示沟之间的牙体组织，约 1.0mm（图 4-23），功能尖颊斜面预备完成后（图 4-24），仍保留原有牙尖解剖轮廓。然后沿着功能尖舌斜面牙尖起伏走行，均匀磨除深度指示沟之间的牙体组织，约 1.0mm（图 4-25），完成功能尖颊舌斜面的预备。

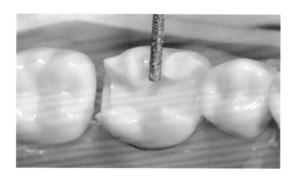

图 4-22 功能尖舌斜面深度指示沟预备

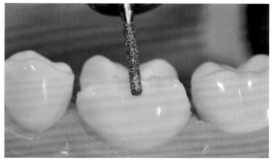

图 4-23 磨除颊斜面深度指示沟之间牙体组织

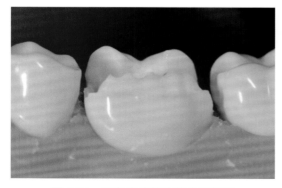

图 4-24 预备完成的功能尖颊斜面

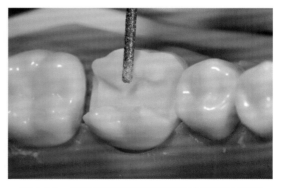

图 4-25 磨除舌斜面深度指示沟之间牙体组织

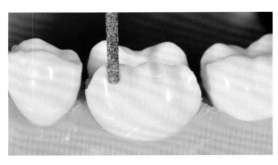 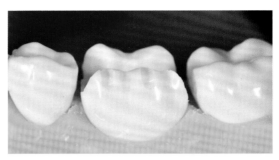

Fig 4-20 The preparation of depth grooves on functional cusp buccal slope of mandibular posterior tooth

Fig 4-21 The preparation of depth grooves on functional cusp buccal slope of mandibular posterior tooth is finished

The same bur is used along the lingual slope of the functional cusps to make 3-4 depth grooves as the methods mentioned above(Fig 4-22). They are 1.0mm deep, exactly the full diameter of the bur inserted into the tooth.

After the preparation of depth grooves on buccal and lingual slope of the functional cusp, the same bur removes the tissue between the grooves uniformly along the buccal slope of the functional cusp, which is about 1.0mm thick (Fig 4-23). The preparation of the buccal inclination on the functional cusps is finished(Fig 4-24), which keeps the original anatomical contour of the cusp. Then removes the tissue between the grooves along the lingual inclination of the functional cusps, which is around 1.0mm(Fig 4-25). The preparation of buccal and lingual inclinations on functional cusp is finished.

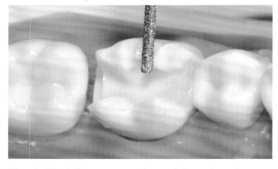 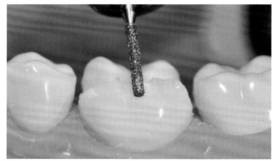

Fig 4-22 The preparation of functional cusp depth grooves on lingual slope

Fig 4-23 Remove the tissue between the depth grooves on buccal slope of functional cusp

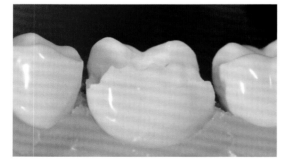 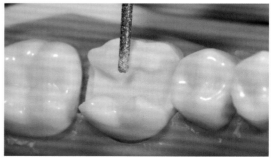

Fig 4-24 The finished preparation of the buccal slope of functional cusp

Fig 4-25 Remove the tissue between the grooves on lingual slope

按照预备功能牙尖的方法，使用同一车针在非功能尖首先预备 3 ～ 4 条深度指示沟（图 4-26）。然后沿着非功能尖牙尖起伏走行，均匀磨除深度指示沟之间的牙体组织（图 4-27），完成非功能尖预备，仍保留非功能尖的解剖轮廓。

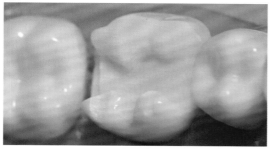
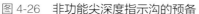
图 4-26　非功能尖深度指示沟的预备

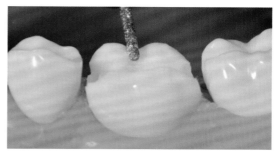
图 4-27　磨除非功能尖深度指示沟之间的牙体组织

为了使高嵌体在功能尖的位置获得足够的支持，需在功能尖颊斜面与颊侧轴面交界的位置预备殆台，方法如下：使用同一车针在下颌后牙功能尖颊斜面与颊轴面交界处预备宽度为 1.0mm 的殆台（图 4-28），车针方向与牙体长轴平行，殆台近远中分别与近远中轴面边缘线贯通，并且实现移行过渡。

预备完成的下颌后牙牙尖殆面观，黄色标记线为殆台（图 4-29）。

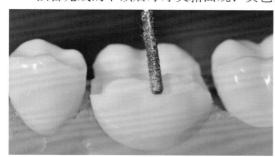
图 4-28　殆台的预备

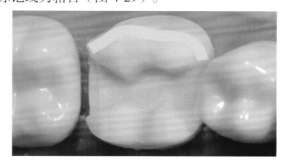
图 4-29　殆台

磨牙高嵌体牙
尖预备

三、精修与磨光

为了获得更加清晰、准确的印模，应对预备体进行精修。此步仅对预备体做磨光处理，不再增加预备量。

使用细粒度的平头圆角锥状金刚砂车针将预备体殆面洞轴壁、各边缘、内线角修整圆钝、光滑（图 4-30）。然后分别磨光近远中邻面箱状洞形的轴壁，使内线角圆钝（图 4-31、图 4-32），做到底平壁直。

Make 3-4 depth grooves on the unfunctional cusps as the methods about preparation of functional cusp by the same bur (Fig 4-26). Remove the tissue uniformly between the depth grooves along the nonfunctional cusps undulated contour(Fig 4-27). The preparation of non-functional cusp is finished, which keeps the original anatomical contour of the nonfunctional cusp.

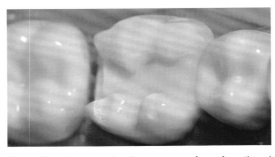 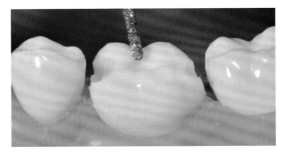

Fig 4-26　Prepare depth grooves of nonfunctional cusp

Fig 4-27　Remove the tissue between the depth grooves on nonfunctional cusp

To gain enough support on functional cusp of the onlay, we prepare the occlusal step on the junction of buccal slope and buccal axial surface of the functional cusp as the following methods: the same bur is used to prepare a 1.0mm wide occlusal step on the junction of buccal slope and buccal axial surface of the functional cusp(Fig 4-28), parallel to the long axial of the tooth. The occlusal step connects with the distal and mesial axial surface margin line and transits naturally.

The occlusal view of the finished mandibular posterior tooth. Yellow line is the outline of the occlusal step(Fig 4-29).

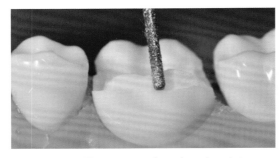 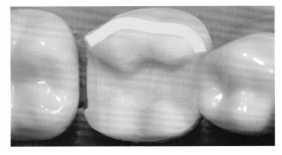

Fig 4-28　The preparation of occlusal step

Fig 4-29　Occlusal step

3. Fine Trimming and Polishing

To gain the impression more clearly, we trim the preparation. This step needs to polish the tooth merely without increasing the reduction.

Using the fine-grained round-end tapered diamond to trim axial walls of occlusal box, margin line, internal corner to be smooth and round(Fig 4-30). Then polish the axial walls of the mesiodistal proximal box to make the internal corner round(Fig 4-31, Fig 4-32). The bottom is flat and the walls are vertical.

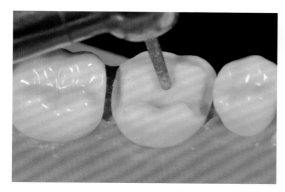

图 4-30　𬌗面洞形的磨光

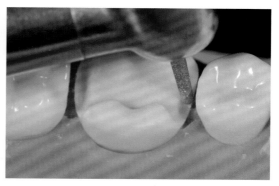

图 4-31　近中邻面洞形的磨光

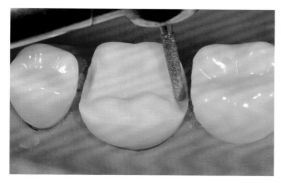

图 4-32　远中邻面洞形的磨光

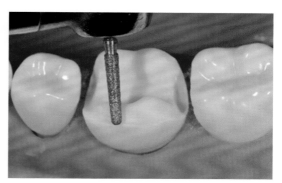

图 4-33　功能尖及𬌗台的磨光

然后对功能尖颊舌斜面及𬌗台（图 4-33）、舌侧非功能尖（图 4-34）进行磨光处理，同时使所有边缘线平缓移行过渡。

如果非功能尖有足够厚（≥ 2.0mm）的牙体组织，可以在非功能尖舌轴面转角处预备非功能尖反斜面，方法如下：在非功能尖预备宽度约 1.0mm、与牙长轴呈 45° 的反斜面（图 4-35），以获得更强的机械固位和更理想的美学效果。

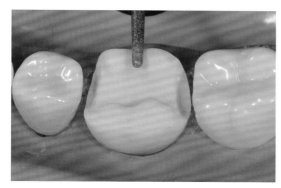

图 4-34　非功能尖的磨光

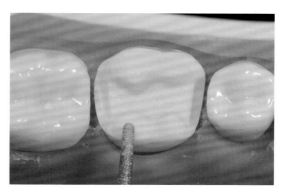

图 4-35　非功能尖反斜面的预备

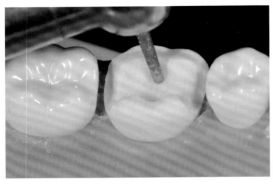

Fig 4-30　Polish the occlusal box

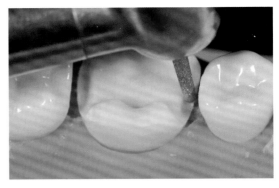

Fig 4-31　Polish the mesial proximal box

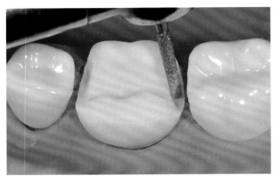

Fig 4-32　Polish the distal proximal box

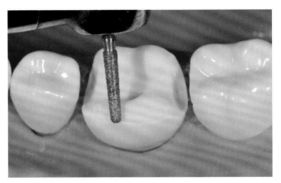

Fig 4-33　Polish the functional cusp and the occlusal step

Then polish the functional cusp buccal and lingual bevels，occlusal step(Fig 4-33) and the lingual nonfunctional cusp(Fig 4-34)，and make the marginal line smooth and move naturally.

If the tissue on nonfunctional cusp is thick enough(≥2mm)，prepare the reverse bevel of nonfunctional cusp on the lingual axial surface of this cusp as the following methods：make a 1.0mm wide bevel on nonfunctional cusp at a 45° with the tooth axial(Fig 4-35) to acquire stronger mechanical retention，achieve better esthetics.

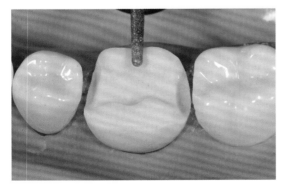

Fig 4-34　Polish the nonfunctional cusp

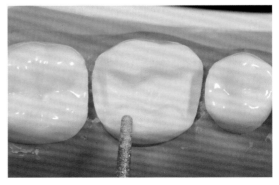

Fig4-35　Prepare a reverse bevel on nonfunctional cusp

最后使用锐利的边缘修整器械修整近中龈壁边缘线（图4-36A）、远中龈壁边缘线（图4-36B）、殆台边缘线，使边缘线光滑、连续，消除飞边（图4-36C），与近远中边缘移行贯通，完成规范的磨牙高嵌体牙体预备。

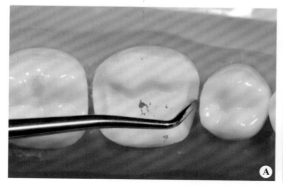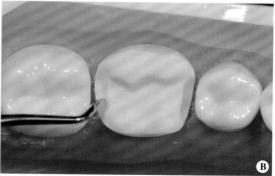

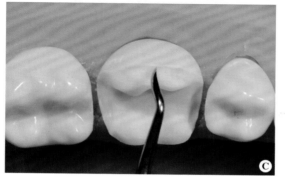

图 4-36　锐利边缘修整器械修整边缘线

高嵌体精修与
磨光

四、高嵌体预备完成

牙体预备完成殆面观（图4-37），洞形底平壁直，内线角圆钝，黄色标线为功能尖殆台。
牙体预备完成舌面观（图4-38），黄色标线为非功能尖反斜面。

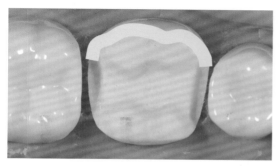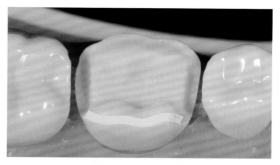

图 4-37　殆面观　　　　　　　　　图 4-38　舌面观

Finally use the sharp edge trimmer to trim the mesial gingival wall margin(Fig 4-36A)，the distal gingival wall margin(Fig 4-36B)，the occlusal step margin to get the margin line smooth and continuous，remove the flash(Fig 4-36C)，which connects to the mesiodistal margin line naturally，then the onlay preparation of posterior tooth is finished.

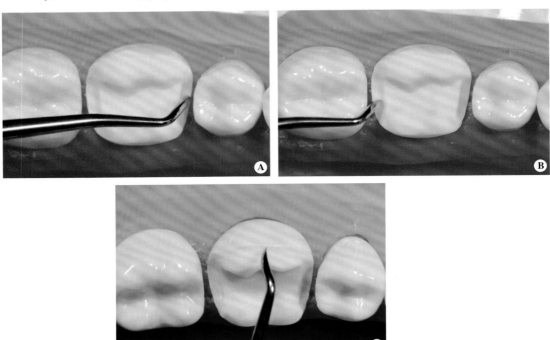

Fig 4-36　Use the sharp fringe trimmer to trim margin line

4. Onlay Preparation is Finished

The occlusal view of the finished preparation(Fig 4-37). The bottom is flat and the walls are vertical with the round internal corner. The yellow line is the occlusal step of the functional cusp.

The lingual view of the finished preparation(Fig 4-38). The yellow line is the opposite area of the nonfunctional cusp.

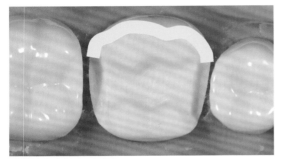

Fig 4-37　The occlusal view

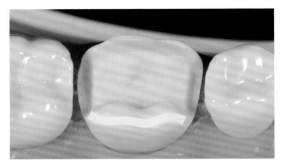

Fig 4-38　The lingual view

第五章 后牙全瓷冠牙体预备

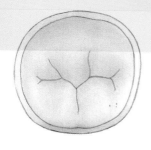

全冠是牙体缺损修复治疗中适应范围最广的一种修复体，覆盖整个缺损患牙的所有轴面和𬌗面，可以用来最大程度地修复缺损患牙的形态、功能，并恢复其美观，还可以用作固定义齿的固位体。全冠按照材料分类大体可以分为金属全冠、金属烤瓷全冠及全瓷冠。

随着生活水平的不断提高，人们对牙冠的美学性能也提出了更高的要求，不仅是前牙全冠，对后牙冠美观性能的关注度也逐步提高，后牙的全瓷冠修复体在临床的应用也越来越广泛。本章就经典的双层结构（氧化锆＋饰瓷）后牙全瓷冠牙体预备做示教，如果是做单层结构的全解剖氧化锆全瓷冠可适当减少预备量，实现微创预备，预备方法相同。后牙全瓷冠牙体预备及预备量见图 5-1。

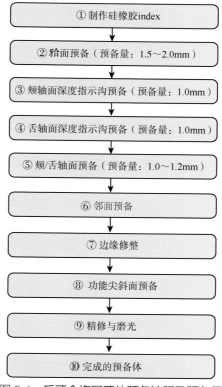

图 5-1　后牙全瓷冠牙体预备流程及预备量

Chapter 5   All-Ceramic Crown Preparation of Posterior Tooth

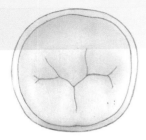

The full crown is the most popular type of crown used in the restoration of dental defects. It covers all the axial and occlusal surfaces of the defected tooth. It can effectively maximize the repair appearance, function and aesthetic of the defected tooth, especially as the retainer of the fixed partial denture. The full crown is classified by the different materials for full crowns, including metal crowns, metal porcelain crowns, and all-ceramic crowns.

As living standard improves, people put forward higher demands for crown esthetics, not only the anterior tooth, but the posterior tooth get more attention about the esthetics performance, and the posterior tooth all-ceramic crown is more and more popular in clinic application. This chapter describes the principles of all-ceramic (zirconia fused porcelain) crown preparation. If the all ceramic crown is monolayer zirconia with anatomical structure, it can reduce the amount of the preparation moderately to achieve minimally invasive preparation, the method is the same. The process of all-ceramic crown posterior preparation and reduction is shown in Fig 5-1.

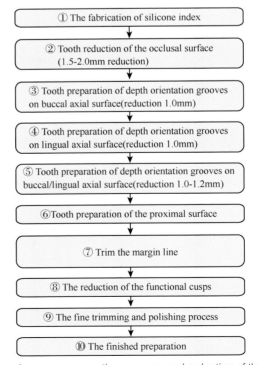

Fig 5-1   All-ceramic crown preparation process and reduction of the posterior tooth

一、制作硅橡胶 index

牙体预备之前使用加成反应硅橡胶油泥混合型制作 index（图 5-2），范围包括预备牙近远中至少两颗牙。

做好的 index 沿预备牙体𬌗面中央做颊舌向垂直切口，切断整个 index（图 5-3）。完成的 index（图 5-4）能暴露出半颗预备牙。

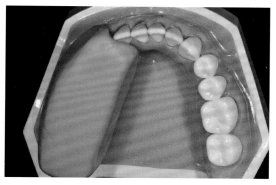

图 5-2　制作 index

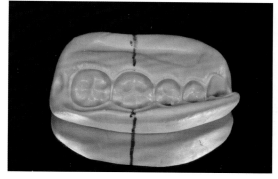

图 5-3　切断 index

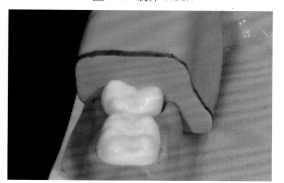

图 5-4　完成的 index

二、𬌗面预备

磨牙的解剖结构比较复杂，𬌗面更是沟窝尖嵴交错纵横，为了能使全瓷冠在𬌗面也能呈现出这样的生理形态，对牙体预备提出了很高的要求，规范的磨牙全瓷冠预备完成后，仍应完全顺应天然磨牙原有的解剖轮廓外形。磨牙全瓷冠𬌗面预备应按照深度指示沟预备及指示沟间牙体组织磨除两个步骤进行。

首先是𬌗面深度指示沟预备。使用直径 1.4mm 的圆角柱状金刚砂车针在颊尖三角嵴顶沿三角嵴走行切入牙体组织，深度 1.4mm，恰好相当于一根车针的直径（图 5-5）。图 5-6 为完成的𬌗面颊侧三角嵴顶深度指示沟。

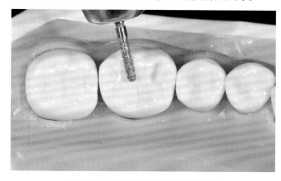

图 5-5　𬌗面深度指示沟预备

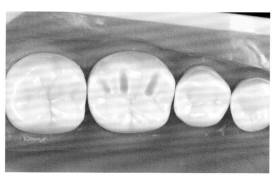

图 5-6　完成的三角嵴顶深度指示沟

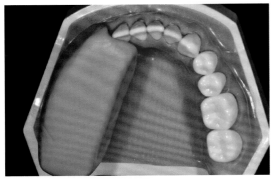

Fig 5-2　Fabricate the index

1. Fabrication of Silicone Index

Before the tooth preparation, the addition type silicone putty is adapted to fabricate a silicone index(Fig 5-2), which covers at least two other adjacent teeth.

The index is sectioned vertically on the center of occlusal surface along the buccal lingual direction of the tooth, which cuts off the whole index(Fig 5-3). The finished index(Fig 5-4) can expose a half bulk of the prepared tooth.

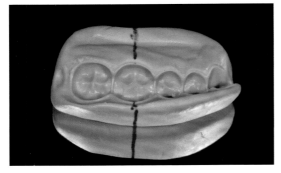

Fig 5-3　Cut off the index

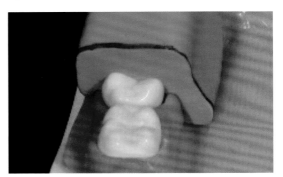

Fig 5-4　The finished index

2. Preparation of Occlusal Surface

The anatomical structure of the posterior tooth is complex particular in the occlusal surface, where the groove, fossa, cusp and ridge distribute crossly. It brings forward high request for preparation. The contour of the all-ceramic crown occlusal surface follows the anatomical form of the natural molar completely. The preparation is separated by two steps: the preparation of the depth grooves and the removing of the tissue.

The first is the occlusal surface depth grooves preparation. Use a 1.4mm diameter round-end tapered diamond bur. The bur is sunk into tissue along the triangular ridge on the buccal triangular ridge, which is 1.4mm deep, exactly equals to a full diameter of the bur(Fig 5-5). Fig 5-6 shows the depth grooves on the buccal triangular ridge of the occlusal surface.

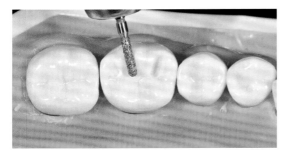

Fig 5-5　Prepare the occlusal depth grooves

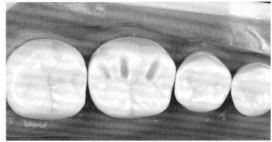

Fig 5-6　The depth grooves of triangular ridge top are finished

　　然后使用同一车针在颊尖三角嵴沟底沿窝沟走行磨入牙体组织（图5-7），深度1.4mm，恰好相当于一根车针的直径，图5-8为完成的𬌗面颊尖三角嵴沟底深度指示沟。只有将深度指示沟定在了三角嵴顶及沟底，在磨除指示沟之间牙体组织时，才能最大限度地沿着磨牙𬌗面解剖外形均匀磨除，从而保证预备完成后𬌗面仍可以保留原有的𬌗面解剖轮廓。

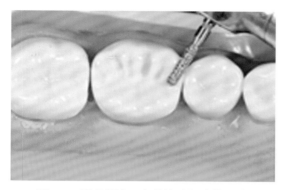

图 5-7　预备颊尖三角嵴沟底深度指示沟

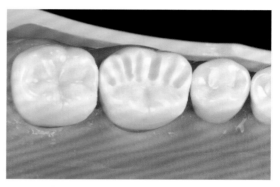

图 5-8　完成的𬌗面颊尖深度指示沟

　　按照相同的方法，使用同一车针在舌尖三角嵴顶沿着三角嵴走行磨入牙体组织（图5-9），深度1.4mm，相当于一根车针的直径，图5-10为完成的𬌗面舌尖三角嵴顶深度指示沟，同样在舌尖三角嵴沟底磨入一根车针的深度（图5-11），这样就完成了𬌗面颊舌牙尖的深度指示沟的预备（图5-12），指示沟分别位于牙尖三角嵴顶和沟底。

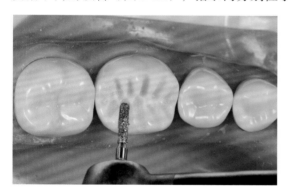

图 5-9　预备舌尖三角嵴顶深度指示沟

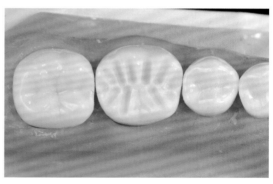

图 5-10　完成的𬌗面舌尖三角嵴顶深度指示沟

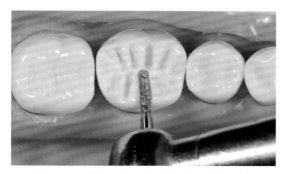

图 5-11　预备舌尖三角嵴沟底深度指示沟

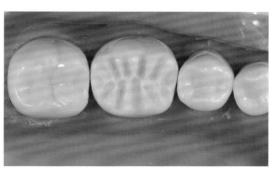

图 5-12　完成的𬌗面深度指示沟

Use the same bur to cut into the tissue following the pits and grooves on the bottom of the grooves between the buccal cusp triangular ridges(Fig 5-7)，the reduction is 1.4mm deep，as the diameter of the bur. Fig 5-8 shows the finished depth grooves on the bottom of the grooves between the buccal cusp triangular ridges of the occlusal surface. Only if the depth grooves locate in the triangular ridge and grooves bottom，the bur can move along the anatomical contour to remove the tissue between the depth grooves uniformly，and the preparation would appear the original anatomical occlusal contour .

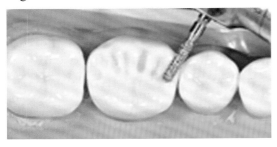

Fig 5-7　Prepare the depth grooves on the bottom of the grooves between the buccal cusp triangular ridges

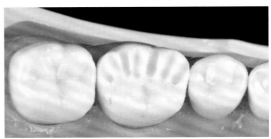

Fig 5-8　The grooves on buccal cusp of occlusal surface are finished

The same bur is sunk into the tissue along the triangular ridge on lingual cusp(Fig 5-9). The grooves are 1.4mm deep，similar equivalent to one bur diameter. Fig 5-10 shows the finished depth grooves on the lingual triangular ridges of occlusal surface. The bur is sunk into the bottom of the triangular ridge groove on lingual cusp(Fig 5-11). In this way，the preparation of buccal and lingual cusp depth groove is finished(Fig 5-12). The depth grooves locate in the triangular ridge top and groove bottom.

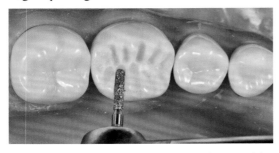

Fig 5-9　Prepare the depth grooves on the top of the lingual cusp triangular ridges

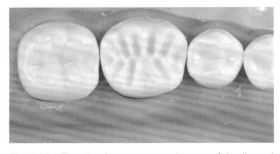

Fig 5-10　The depth grooves on the top of the lingual cusp triangular ridges are finished

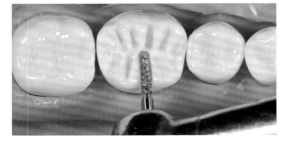

Fig 5-11　Prepare the depth grooves on the bottom of the grooves between the lingual cusp triangular ridges

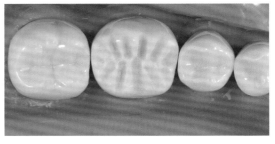

Fig 5-12　The finished occlusal surface depth grooves

　　𬌗面牙尖深度指示沟预备完成后，分别沿牙尖嵴斜面走行及磨牙𬌗面解剖形态逐步均匀磨除指示沟间的牙体组织。

　　首先磨除颊尖深度指示沟间的牙体组织，车针分别沿颊尖每个三角嵴斜面走行，从每一条三角嵴顶的指示沟分别向近远中方向均匀磨除牙体组织至三角嵴沟底的指示沟。在近远中边缘嵴处应尽量越过近远中边缘嵴，应避免伤及邻牙（图5-13）。

　　此时需强调一点，在磨除指示沟间牙体组织时，预备在𬌗面中央沟底应有重叠和交叉，以保证在中央沟也有足量的预备。完成的颊尖三角嵴预备（图5-14），颊尖𬌗面形态仍保留原牙的𬌗面颊尖解剖轮廓。

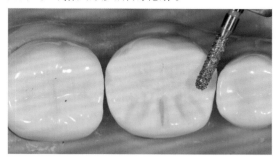
图5-13　车针沿着颊尖三角嵴预备

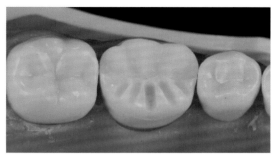
图5-14　完成的颊尖三角嵴预备

　　按照上述方法，使用同一车针在舌尖三角嵴逐步磨除舌尖深度指示沟之间的牙体组织（图5-15），近远中需越过边缘嵴（图5-16），预备时避免伤及邻牙。在磨除指示沟间牙体组织时，预备𬌗面中央沟底应与颊尖预备部分有重叠和交叉，以保证在中央沟也有足量的预备。

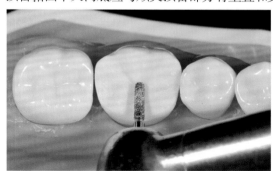
图5-15　磨除舌尖深度指示沟间的牙体组织

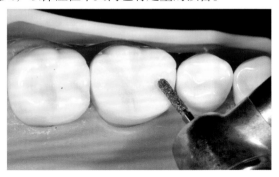
图5-16　预备越过边缘嵴

　　预备完成的𬌗面牙尖三角嵴（图5-17），形态仍保留原牙的𬌗面解剖轮廓。

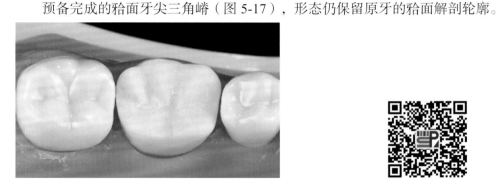
图5-17　𬌗面预备完成，形态仍保留原牙轮廓

磨牙全瓷冠𬌗面预备

Remove the tissue gradually between the grooves along the cusp ridge slope and anatomical contour of occlusal surface uniformly after the preparation of the depth grooves on occlusal cusp.

Remove the tissue between the buccal grooves firstly，the bur moves along the buccal cusp triangular ridge slope towards mesiodistal to prepare from the triangular ridge top depth groove to the bottom one evenly. Try to cross the mesial and distal marginal ridge without damage to adjacent tooth(Fig 5-13).

It is emphasized that the overlapping and cross section of the removing is needed in bottom of the central sulcus on occlusal surface when we remove the tissue between the depth grooves，which ensures enough reduction here. The preparation of buccal cusp is finished(Fig 5-14). The reduction follows the outline of the unprepared buccal cusp contours.

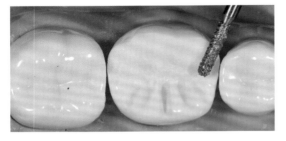
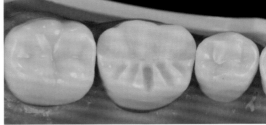

Fig 5-13　The bar follows along the slope of the buccal cusp triangular ridge

Fig5-14　The preparation of buccal cusp is finished

The tissue between the depth grooves of lingual cusp from triangular ridge of lingual cusps is gradually removed(Fig 5-15)，which crosses the mesialdistal marginal ridges(Fig 5-16). Be careful not to damage the adjacent tooth. It is emphasized that the overlapping and crossing section of the removing is needed in central sulcus of occlusal surface when we remove the tissue between the depth grooves，which ensures enough reduction here.

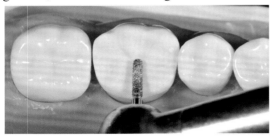

Fig 5-15　The tissue between the depth grooves of lingual cusp is removed

Fig 5-16　The preparation crosses the marginal ridge

The preparation of triangular ridge on occlusal cusp is finished(Fig 5-17). The preparation keeps the outline of the original anatomical contours.

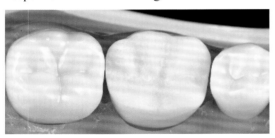

Fig 5-17　The finished occlusal surface keeps the outline of the original anatomical contours

三、颊轴面深度指示沟预备

　　𬌗面预备完成后进行的是颊舌轴面预备，首先是颊轴面的预备。按照下颌磨牙的解剖外形，颊轴面也分为两个轴面，即𬌗 2/3 轴面与颈 1/3 轴面预备。

　　使用直径 1.0mm 的圆头柱状金刚砂车针，分别在𬌗 2/3 和颈 1/3 切入牙体组织，没入一根车针的量，完成 1.0mm 深度指示沟的预备，应分别在牙体颊轴面最凸和最凹的位置预备深度指示沟（图 5-18），颈 1/3 的深度指示沟也是如此（图 5-19）。

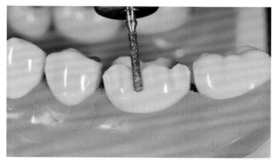
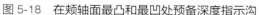

图 5-18　在颊轴面最凸和最凹处预备深度指示沟

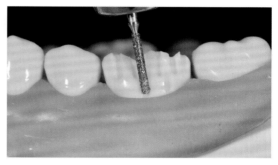

图 5-19　颈 1/3 的深度指示沟

　　两个部分的深度指示沟车针放置方向分别与𬌗 2/3 轴面平行（图 5-20）、颈 1/3 轴面平行（图 5-21）。

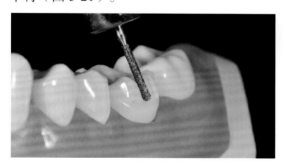

图 5-20　车针与𬌗 2/3 轴面平行

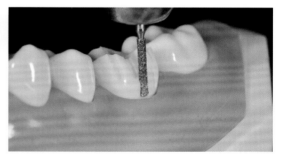

图 5-21　车针与颈 1/3 轴面平行

　　颊轴面深度指示沟预备完成（图 5-22）。两部分的指示沟在颊轴面外形高点线处应相互重叠。

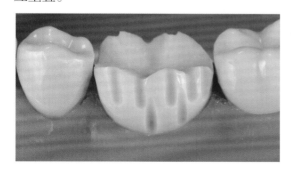

图 5-22　颊轴面深度指示沟预备完成

颊轴面深度指示沟预备

3. Preparation of Depth Grooves on Buccal Axial Surface

Prepare the buccal and lingual axial surface after the preparation of occlusal surface. Firstly prepare the buccal axial surface according to the anatomical contour of mandibular molars, which is separated by two parts: occlusal 2/3 axial surface and cervical 1/3 axial surface.

Cut into the tissue on the occlusal 2/3 and the cervical 1/3 planes by using a 1.0mm diameter round-end tapered diamond. The grooves are produced 1.0mm deep as a diameter of the bur on the most convex and concave part of the buccal plane(Fig 5-18). The grooves on the buccal cervical 1/3 surface is the same(Fig 5-19).

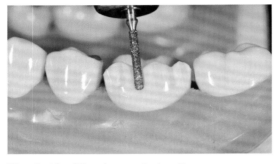 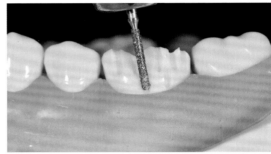

Fig 5-18 The buccal depth grooves are prepared on the most convex and concave part

Fig 5-19 The depth grooves on the buccal cervical 1/3 surface

The bur direction of two parts is parallel to the occlusal 2/3 axial surface(Fig 5-20) and cervical 1/3 axial surface respectively(Fig 5-21).

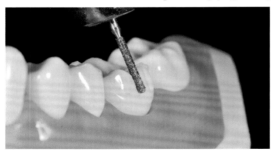 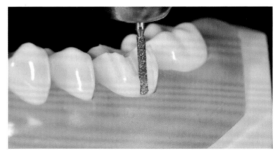

Fig 5-20 The bur is parallel to the uncut occlusal 2/3 axial surface

Fig 5-21 The bur parallels the uncut cervical 1/3 axial surface

The grooves on buccal surface are finished(Fig 5-22). The grooves of two parts overlap on the height line of contour.

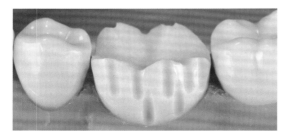

Fig 5-22 The depth grooves on buccal surface are finished

四、舌轴面深度指示沟预备

使用直径 1.0mm 的圆头柱状金刚砂车针沿与舌轴面平行的方向切入牙体组织，深度 1.0mm，相当于一根车针的直径，应分别在牙体舌轴面最凸和最凹的位置制备深度指示沟（图 5-23）。

完成的舌轴面深度指示沟见图 5-24。

颊舌轴面深度指示沟预备完成，𬌗面观（图 5-25），指示沟的方向顺应下颌磨牙的解剖外形，深度为均匀的 1.0mm。为了防止预备过量，可以在指示沟底涂上颜色标记，在精修与磨光之前此颜色标记不能消除。

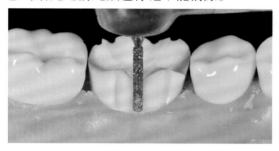

图 5-23　在牙体舌轴面最凸和最凹的位置制备深度指示沟

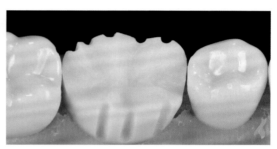

图 5-24　舌轴面深度指示沟完成

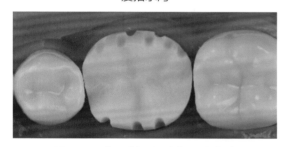

图 5-25　颊舌轴面深度指示沟完成

舌轴面深度指示沟预备

五、颊舌轴面预备

下一步是按照颊舌轴面深度指示沟指示的深度磨除指示沟间的牙体组织。首先是颊面指示沟间的牙体组织磨除，仍需按𬌗 2/3 和颈 1/3 两个轴面分别进行。

使用直径 1.4mm 的圆头柱状金刚砂车针顺应颊面解剖形态磨除𬌗 2/3 深度指示沟之间的牙体组织（图 5-26），磨除时车针放置方向与𬌗 2/3 轴面平行，沿下颌磨牙颊面起伏走行预备，近远中尽量向邻接区扩展（图 5-27），以最大程度减少打开邻接时的阻力，切勿伤及邻牙。

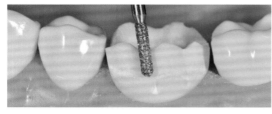

图 5-26　磨除颊面𬌗 2/3 深度指示沟之间的牙体组织

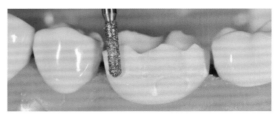

图 5-27　近远中尽量向邻接区扩展

4. Preparation of Depth Grooves on Lingual Axial Surface

Using a 1.0mm diameter round-end tapered diamond to cut into the tooth tissue in a direction parallel to the lingual axial surface. The depth is 1.0mm, as a diameter of a bur, prepare the grooves on the most convex and concave part of the lingual axial plane respectively(Fig 5-23).

The depth grooves on lingual surface is finished(Fig 5-24).

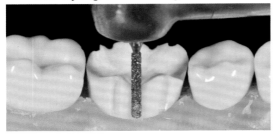

Fig 5-23   Prepare the depth grooves on the most convex and concave part of the lingual axial plane respectively

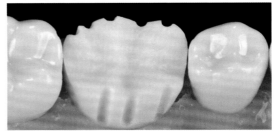

Fig 5-24   The depth grooves on lingual surface are finished

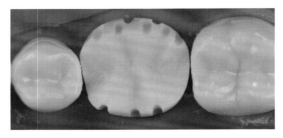

Fig 5-25   The depth grooves on buccal and lingual axial surface are finished

The depth grooves on buccal and lingual axial surfaces are finished. On the occlusal view (Fig 5-25). The direction of the depth grooves follows the anatomical contour of the posterior tooth, the depth is 1.0mm evenly. Color the bottom of the depth grooves as marks, which should not be removed before the fine trimming and polishing process to prevent preparing too much tooth.

5. Preparation of Buccal and Lingual Surfaces

Next is to remove the tissue between the depth grooves on buccal and lingual axial surface. Firstly, remove the tissue between grooves on buccal surface, which is performed as occlusal 2/3 and cervical 1/3 two parts.

Replace the bur by a 1.4mm diameter round-end tapered diamond. Following the contour of the buccal shape, the tissue between the depth grooves of the occlusal 2/3 surface is removed(Fig 5-26). The bur is parallel to the occlusal 2/3 axial surface, which is swept across the buccal surface along the undulant contour of the buccal surface as far into the facial embrasures as possible (Fig 5-27), so that it can reduce drag of opening the contact. Take care not to damage the adjacent tooth.

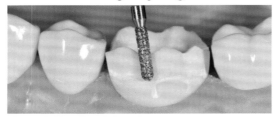

Fig 5-26   The tissue between the depth grooves is removed

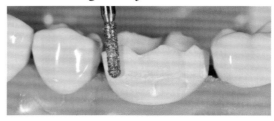

Fig 5-27   The mesiodistal preparation extends as far into the contact area

殆面 2/3 深度指示沟之间的牙体组织磨除完成，颊面观（图 5-28），仍可见到牙尖轮廓形态；殆面观（图 5-29），预备后仍保留颊轴面起伏的外形。

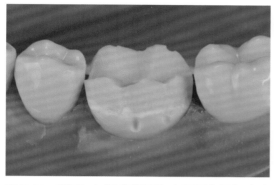

图 5-28　殆面 2/3 深度指示沟之间牙体组织磨除完成，颊面观

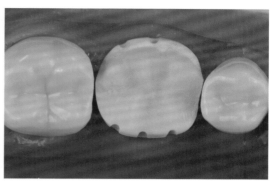

图 5-29　殆面观

使用同一车针顺应颊面解剖形态磨除颈 1/3 深度指示沟之间的牙体组织，同时在颈部形成边缘线（图 5-30）。车针放置方向与颈 1/3 轴面平行，预备近远中轴角时尽量向邻面外展隙扩展（图 5-31），避免伤及邻牙。

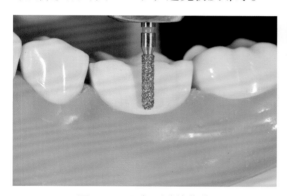

图 5-30　颈部形成边缘线

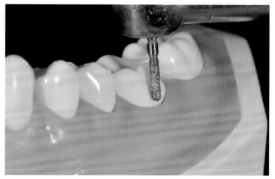

图 5-31　预备近远中轴角时尽量向邻面外展隙扩展

颊轴面预备完成后，因牙体组织被磨除了 1.0mm 左右厚度，在颈部齐龈位置会形成宽 1.0mm、内线角圆钝的颊侧边缘线，完全顺应龈缘走行（图 5-32）。

殆面观，仍保留原牙颊轴面的解剖轮廓（图 5-33）。

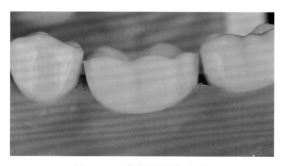

图 5-32　颊轴面预备完成

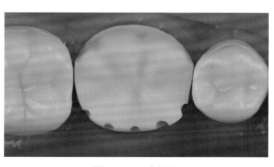

图 5-33　殆面观

The tissue between the depth grooves on occlusal 2/3 of buccal surface is removed. The buccal view(Fig 5-28) still retains the contour of the cusps. And the occlusal view(Fig 5-29) keeps the waved contour of the buccal axial surface.

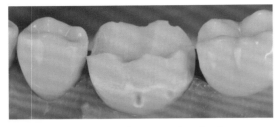

Fig 5-28　The tissues between the depth grooves on occlusal 2/3 buccal surface is removed

Fig 5-29　The occlusal view

The tissue between the depth grooves of the cervical 1/3 surface is removed by following the contour of the buccal surface shape(Fig 5-30). The bur is parallel to the cervical 1/3 axial surface(Fig 5-31). The mesialdistal axial angle preparation extends as far into the proximal embrasures as possible without damage to the adjacent teeth.

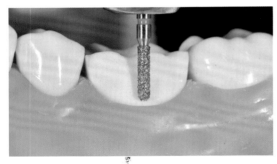
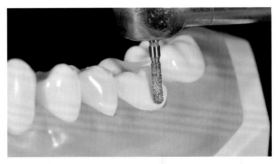

Fig 5-30　Cervical margin line is finished

Fig 5-31　The mesialdistal axial angle preparation extends as far into the proximal embrasures as possible

The buccal surface preparation is finished. The reduction is about 1.0mm so that a 1.0mm wide buccal margin line with a rounded internal angle can be formed，which follows the direction of the gingival edge(Fig 5-32).

On the occlusal view，the preparation keeps the anatomical contour of the buccal axial surface(Fig 5-33).

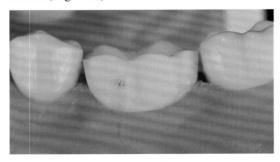
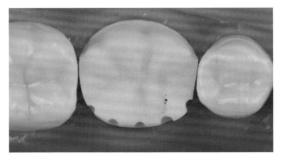

Fig 5-32　The buccal surface preparation is finished

Fig 5-33　The occlusal view

　　使用同一车针按照磨除颊轴面深度指示沟间牙体组织的方法逐步均匀磨除舌轴面深度指示沟之间的牙体组织（图 5-34），不同的是舌轴面只需按一个面预备即可，应完全顺应舌轴面原来的解剖走行进行预备。

　　舌轴面预备完成（图 5-35），从𬌗面观仍保留舌轴面原来的解剖轮廓外形，同时在颈部形成平齐龈缘处 1.0mm 宽、内线角圆钝的边缘线，完全顺应舌侧龈缘走行，颊舌轴面形成 6°～ 8° 的聚合度，预备尽量向邻接区扩展，避免伤及邻牙。

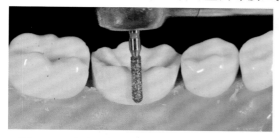

图 5-34　磨除舌轴面深度指示沟间的牙体组织

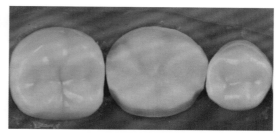

图 5-35　舌轴面预备完成，𬌗面观

　　颊轴面预备完成，颊面观（图 5-36）。

　　舌轴面预备完成，舌面观（图 5-37）。此种预备方法已将邻面牙体组织部分磨除，对于下一步顺利打开邻接奠定了基础。

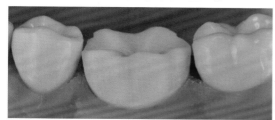

图 5-36　颊轴面预备完成，颊面观

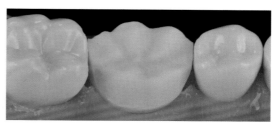

图 5-37　舌轴面预备完成，舌面观

颊舌轴面预备

六、邻面预备

　　此步的预备要点是打开邻接，但不能伤及邻牙，预备方法与前牙全瓷冠打开邻接的方法基本相同。使用细针状金刚砂车针，车针完全没入预备牙近远中边缘嵴，平行于牙长轴，从𬌗面逐步向根方切入（图 5-38），保留预备牙体近远中邻面釉质薄片，这样可最大限度地避免伤及邻牙。

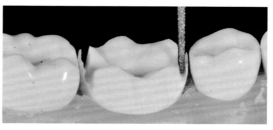

图 5-38　车针平行于牙长轴，从𬌗面逐步向根方切入

111

The tissue between the depth grooves on the lingual axial surface is removed by the same bur as the method of removing the tissue between buccal axial surface depth grooves(Fig 5-34). The preparation follows the original anatomical contour of the lingual surface.

The preparation of lingual surface is finished(Fig 5-35)，which keeps the original anatomical contour on the buccal view. A 1.0mm wide margin line with a round internal angle is formed at the the level of gingival edge following the direction of the lingual gingival margin. It exhibits 6°-8° taper between the buccal and lingual wall. The mesialdistal preparation extends as far into the contact area as possible without damage to the adjacent teeth.

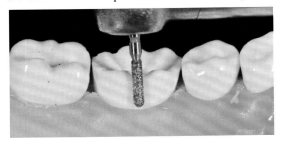

Fig 5-34　Remove the tissue between the depth grooves on lingual axial surface

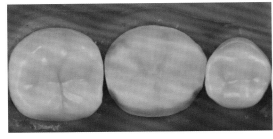

Fig 5-35　The preparation of lingual axial surface is finished

The preparation of buccal axial surface is finished. The buccal view(Fig 5-36).

The preparation of lingual axial surface is finished. The lingual view(Fig 5-37). The preparation method removes the proximal tissue partly，which lays the foundation for next step to open the contact.

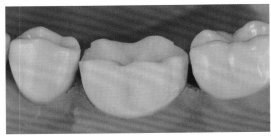
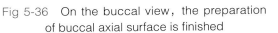

Fig 5-36　On the buccal view，the preparation of buccal axial surface is finished

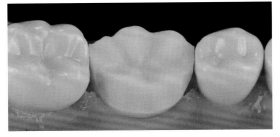

Fig 5-37　On the lingual view，the preparation of lingual axial surface is finished

6. Preparation of Proximal Surface

The key point of the step is opening contact area without damage to the adjacent teeth. The preparation method is same as the all-ceramic crown contact of the anterior tooth. Use a smaller round-end tapered diamond bur to cut into the mesiodistal marginal ridge of the preparation. The bur parallels the long axial of the tooth cutting from the occlusal down to the root gradually(Fig 5-38). In this sequence there are thin enamel chips remaining on the proximal surface so that it can avoid to damage to the adjacent teeth largely.

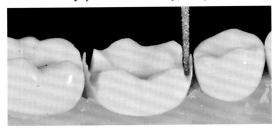

Fig 5-38　The bur parallels the long axial of the tooth cutting from the occlusal down to the root gradually

需强调的是，邻面预备时车针切勿直接进入邻接区（图 5-39），车针与邻牙完全不接触，可以最大程度地保护邻牙。𬌗面观，釉质薄片仍留在预备牙上（图 5-40），继续向根方预备直至薄片脱落，邻接打开。

然后用直径 1.0mm 的圆头柱状金刚砂车针顺应牙体形态，分别从近远中颊侧外展隙进入邻接区已打开的沟槽，并逐步向舌侧磨除（图 5-41），在近远中邻面颈部形成 1.0mm 宽的龈边缘线。

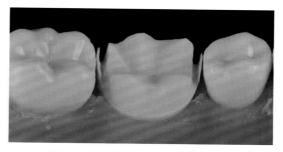

图 5-39 车针切勿直接进入邻接区

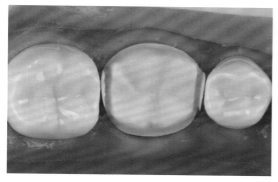

图 5-40 𬌗面观

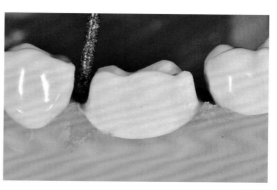

图 5-41 磨除釉质薄片

邻面预备时，车针完全不接触邻牙邻面，避免伤及邻牙（图 5-42）。

邻接完全打开后，形成宽 1.0mm、内线角圆钝的邻面边缘线，位置平齐龈缘（图 5-43），与颊舌侧的边缘线自然移行贯通，完全顺应邻面牙龈乳头缘走行，此时近远中邻面的聚合度不应超过 6°。

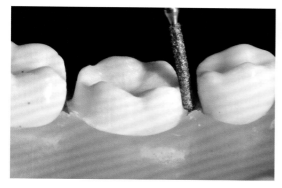

图 5-42 打开邻接

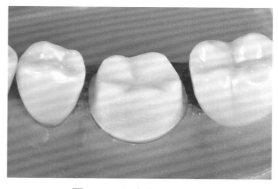

图 5-43 预备邻面边缘线

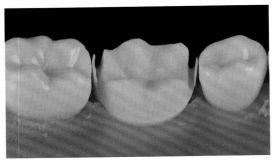

Fig5-39 Forbid entering to the contact area directly

During the preparation process, it needs to be emphasized that forbid entering to the contact area directly. The bur does not contact the adjacent tooth at all to protect the adjacent tooth mostly. The occlusal view. The enamel chips stay in the prepared tooth(Fig 5-40). Keep on preparing towards the root until the chips are removed and the contact is broken.

A 1.0mm diameter round-end tapered diamond gets through the proximal surface from the mesiodistal buccal embrasure to the lingual surface according to the contour of the tooth(Fig 5-41), which forms the 1.0mm wide gingival margin line on mesiodistal cervical part of the proximal surface.

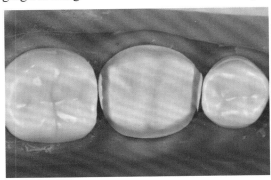

Fig 5-40 The occlusal view

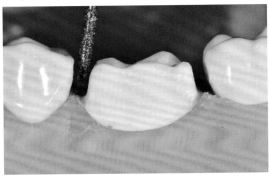

Fig 5-41 Removes the remaining enamel chips

When preparing the proximal surface, we keep the bur out of the adjacent tooth without damage to the adjacent tooth(Fig 5-42).

When the proximal contact is broken, a 1.0mm wide proximal margin line with a round internal angle is formed, which is placed at the level of the gingival margin(Fig 5-43). The margin line connects with the finish lines of buccal and lingual surfaces naturally, following the contour of gingival papilla. Then the taper of the mesiodistal walls is at most 6°.

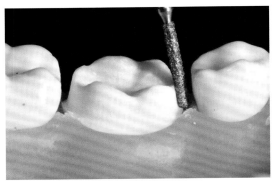

Fig 5-42 The proximal contact is broken

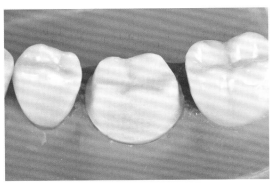

Fig 5-43 Prepare the proximal margin line

邻面预备完成，殆面观（图 5-44），预备体颈部环状边缘线清晰、连续完整。

邻面预备完成，舌面观（图 5-45），边缘线平齐龈缘，顺应龈缘走行。

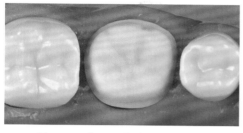

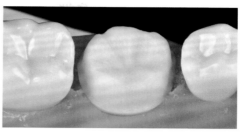

图 5-44　邻面预备完成，殆面观

图 5-45　舌面观

邻面预备

七、边缘修整

接下来进行龈边缘线的修整，对于龈边缘线的要求是：清晰、光滑、连续、完整、顺应龈缘走行。使用直径 1.0mm 的圆头柱状金刚砂车针按照完全顺应牙龈缘走行且平行于牙长轴的方向进行修整，形成宽 1.0mm、内线角圆钝的龈边缘线。

修整龈边缘线从颊侧开始（图 5-46）转向近中（图 5-47）、远中（图 5-48），再分别从近远中转向舌面（图 5-49），使其连续、自然移行过渡，顺应牙龈缘走行。

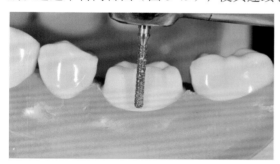

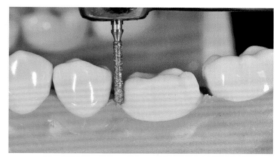

图 5-46　修整颊侧龈边缘线

图 5-47　修整近中龈边缘线

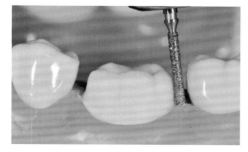

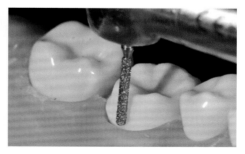

图 5-48　修整远中龈边缘线

图 5-49　修整舌侧龈边缘线

边缘修整

The proximal preparation is finished on the occlusal view(Fig 5-44). The cyclic marginal line on cervical part is clear and continuous.

The proximal preparation is finished on the lingual view(Fig 5-45), the line is at the level of margin following the direction of gingiva.

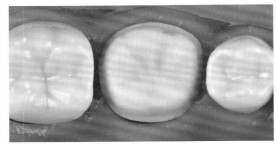

Fig 5-44　The proximal preparation is finished on the occlusal view

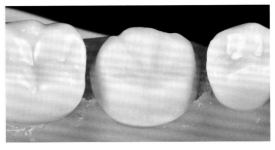

Fig 5-45　The lingual view

7. Trimming the Margin Line

Then, trim the gingival margin line, the demands for the gingival margin line is clear, smooth, continuous, complete and following the gingival margin. The cervical margin line is trimmed with a 1.0mm diameter round-end tapered diamond following the gingival contours, the bur parallels the axial direction. A 1.0mm wide margin line with a rounded internal line angle is formed.

The margin line is trimmed from buccal(Fig 5-46) to the mesial surface(Fig 5-47), and then to the distal surface(Fig 5-48), and from proximal to lingual surface separately(Fig 5-49), which is continuous and transits naturally, following the gingival contours.

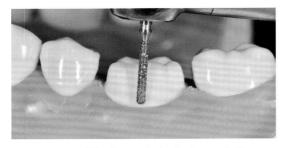

Fig 5-46　Trim buccal gingival margin line

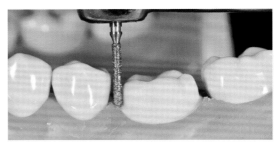

Fig 5-47　Trim mesial gingival margin line

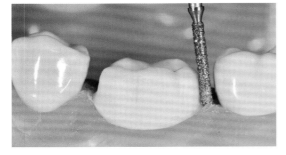

Fig 5-48　Trim distal gingival margin line

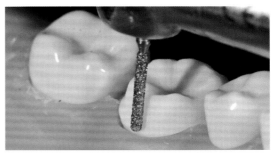

Fig 5-49　Trim lingual gingival margin line

八、功能尖斜面预备

下颌磨牙的颊尖是功能牙尖，颊尖的颊侧斜面要承担较大的咬合应力。此位置对全冠修复体的强度就提出了更高的要求，而修复体强度的决定因素除了材料属性，还取决于修复体材料的厚度。为了能使功能牙尖区的修复体厚度更大，使修复体更坚硬，需在此位置磨除更多的牙体组织，开辟更大的修复体空间，方法是在颊侧牙尖制备功能尖斜面。使用直径 1.4mm 的圆头柱状金刚砂车针沿着功能尖（颊尖）的颊斜面（图 5-50）与牙体长轴约呈 45°（图 5-51），均匀磨除约 1.0mm 厚的牙体组织，形成宽度约 1.5mm 的功能尖斜面。

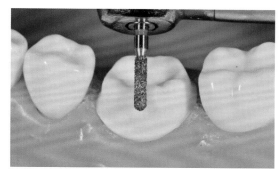

图 5-50　功能尖斜面的位置

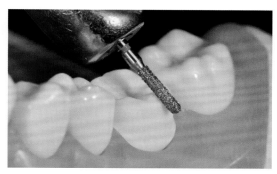

图 5-51　车针与牙体长轴呈 45°

完成的功能尖斜面，颊面观（图 5-52），颜色标记处即功能尖斜面。

完成的功能尖斜面，𬌗面观（图 5-53）。

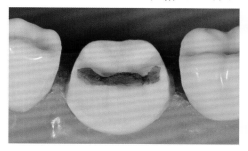

图 5-52　完成的功能尖斜面，颊面观

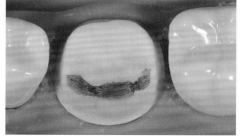

图 5-53　完成的功能尖斜面，𬌗面观

功能尖斜面制备

九、精修与磨光

最后的步骤是精修与磨光，以获得足够清晰的印模和足够好的内冠及边缘适合性。使用直径 1.4mm 的细粒度圆头柱状金刚砂车针将预备体颊轴面（图 5-54）、舌轴面（图 5-55），以及近远中邻面和所有的线角、面角、轴角修整圆钝，磨光预备体。

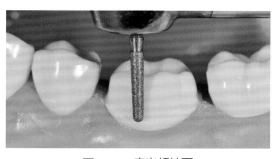

图 5-54　磨光颊轴面

8. Preparation of Functional Cusp Bevel

The functional cusp of the mandibular molar is the buccal cusp, where the buccal bevel bears more occlusal force. This area demands more on the strength of the all-crown restoration. The strength of the restoration derives from the material and the thickness of the material. Grind more teeth in the functional cusp to acquire more place for restoration, in this way, the material is thick enough to be hard. The method is to prepare the functional cusp bevel in buccal cusp. Use a 1.4mm diameter round-end tapered diamond along the functional cusp bevel(Fig 5-50), which is placed to intersect with the tooth axial at the 45° angle(Fig 5-51), remove the 1.0mm tissue evenly, and then creates the 1.5mm wide functional cusp bevel.

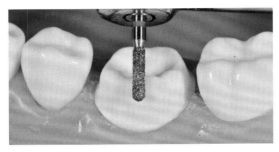

Fig 5-50　The location of the bevel on the functional cusp

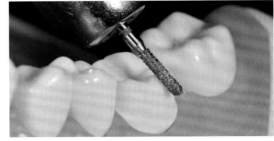

Fig 5-51　The angel between bur and axial of tooth is 45°

The bevel on functional cusp is finished. On the buccal view(Fig 5-52). The marker is the functional cusp bevel.

The bevel on functional cusp is finished. On the occlusal view(Fig 5-53).

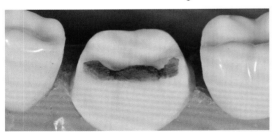

Fig 5-52　The buccal view of the finished functional cusp bevel

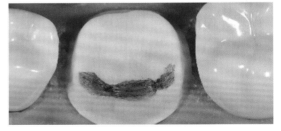

Fig 5-53　The occlusal view of the finished functional cusp bevel

9. Fine Trimming and Polishing

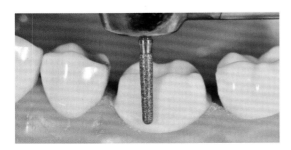

Fig 5-54　Polish the buccal axial surface

Finally, trim and polish the preparation to make the impression more clear, the preparation and the inner crown more dense. Use a 1.4mm diameter fine-grained round-end tapered diamond to smooth and refine the buccal surfaces(Fig 5-54), lingual surface(Fig 5-55), proximal surface, line angles, axial angles and plane angles.

使用同一车针，沿𬌗面原解剖轮廓走行磨光预备体𬌗面（图 5-56）。

使用锐利的边缘修整器械，对颊侧颈部边缘线（图 5-57）、近远中邻面边缘线（图 5-58）及舌侧颈部边缘线（图 5-59）进行光滑处理，消除飞边，使边缘线清晰、光滑连续。

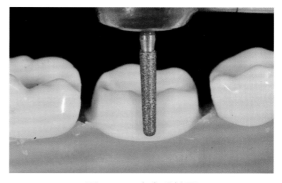

图 5-55　磨光舌轴面

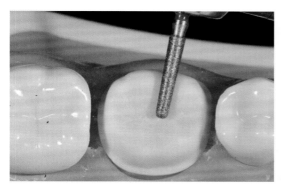

图 5-56　磨光𬌗面

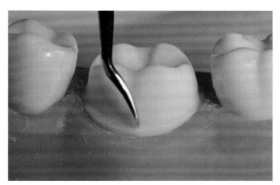

图 5-57　消除颊侧边缘线的飞边

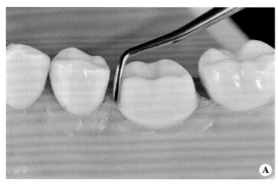

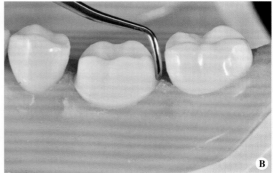

图 5-58　消除近远中邻面边缘线的飞边

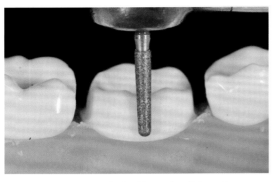

Fig 5-55　Polish the lingual axial surface

Polish the occlusal surface of the preparation along the original anatomical contour by the same bur(Fig 5-56).

The margin line of the cervical buccal surface(Fig 5-57), mesiodistal proximal surface(Fig 5-58) and cervical lingual surface(Fig 5-59) is trimmed smoothly by a sharp fringe trimmer, the flash is removed, which makes the margin line clear, smooth and continuous.

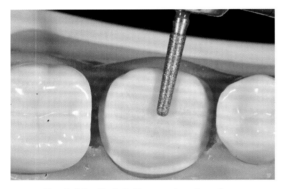

Fig 5-56　Polish the occlusal surface

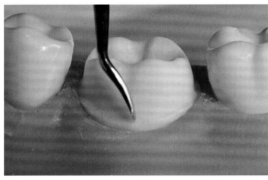

Fig 5-57　Remove the flash of the buccal margin line

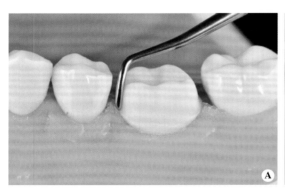

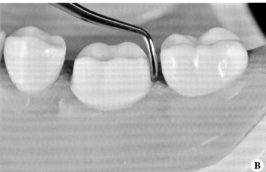

Fig 5-58　Remove the flash of the mesial and distal proximal margin lines

完成的预备体，𬌗面观（图 5-60），保留原来的𬌗面解剖轮廓外形。

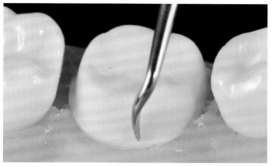

图 5-59　消除舌侧边缘线的飞边

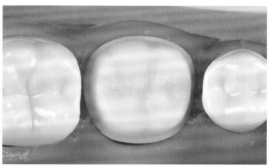

图 5-60　完成的预备体，𬌗面观

完成的预备体，颊面观（图 5-61），保留原来的颊侧解剖轮廓外形。

完成的预备体，舌面观（图 5-62）。

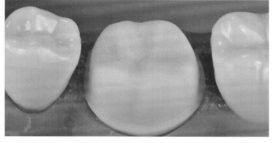

图 5-61　完成的预备体，颊面观

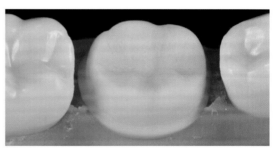

图 5-62　完成的预备体，舌面观

戴入 index，并使用牙周探针检查，可见𬌗面均匀磨除，预备量为 1.5 ～ 2.0mm（图 5-63），颊面亦均匀磨除，预备量为 1.0 ～ 1.2mm（图 5-64），预备体保留原来的解剖轮廓及外形。

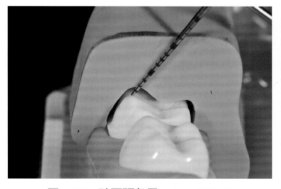

图 5-63　𬌗面预备量 1.5 ～ 2.0mm

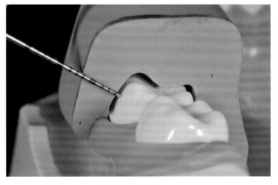

图 5-64　颊面预备量 1.0 ～ 1.2mm

边缘修整

The occlusal view of the finished preparation(Fig 5-60). The shape of the prepared surface follows the contour of the original tooth.

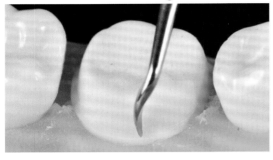

Fig 5-59　Remove the flash of the lingual cervical margin line

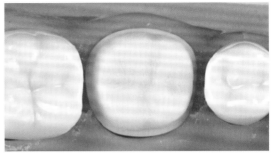

Fig 5-60　The occlusal view of the finished preparation

The buccal view of the finished preparation(Fig 5-61). The shape of the prepared surface follows the contour of the original tooth.

The lingual view of the finished preparation(Fig 5-62).

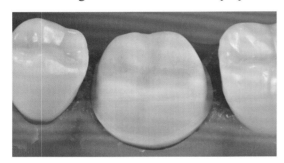

Fig 5-61　The buccal view of the finished preparation

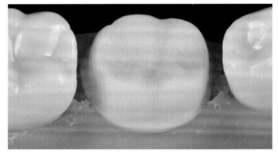

Fig 5-62　The lingual view of the finished preparation

The index is placed over the preparation，and a periodontal probe is placed on the index to show the uniform 1.5-2.0mm occlusal reduction(Fig 5-63)and the 1.0-1.2mm buccal reduction (Fig 5-64). The reduction follows the geometric outline of the occlusal surface.

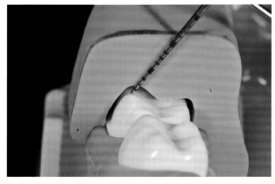

Fig 5-63　1.5-2.0mm reduction on occlusal surface

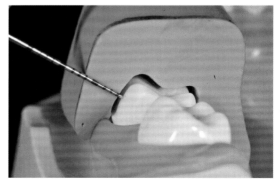

Fig 5-64　1.0-1.2mm reduction on buccal surface

十、完成的预备体

完成的预备体，颊面观（图 5-65）、舌面观（图 5-66）边缘线均平行于釉牙骨质界（牙龈缘）走行，预备体保留原来的解剖轮廓外形，绿色标线为功能尖斜面，蓝色标线为颈部边缘线。

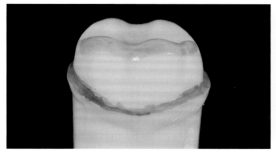

图 5-65　完成的预备体，颊面观

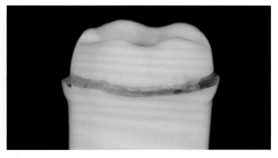

图 5-66　完成的预备体，舌面观

完成的预备体，近中邻面观（图 5-67）、远中邻面观（图 5-68）边缘线均平行于釉牙骨质界（牙龈缘）走行，预备体保留原来的解剖轮廓外形。

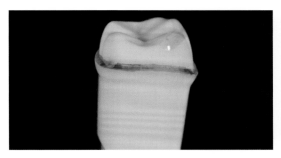

图 5-67　完成的预备体，近中邻面观

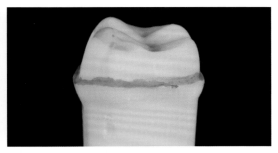

图 5-68　完成的预备体，远中邻面观

完成的预备体，𬌗面观（图 5-69），预备体保留𬌗面原来的解剖轮廓外形。

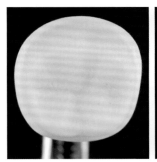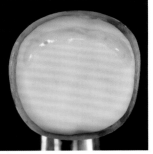

图 5-69　完成的预备体，𬌗面观

10. The Finished Preparation

The buccal view(Fig 5-65) and the lingual view(Fig 5-66) of the finished preparation. The marginal line parallels the direction of the CEJ(cemento-enamel junction). The shape of the prepared surface follows the anatomical contours of the original tooth. The green line is functional cusp bevel, and the blue one is cervical margin line.

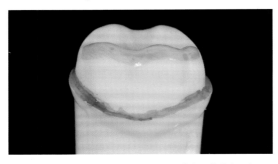 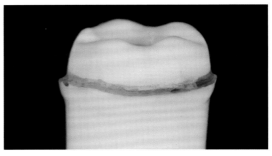

Fig 5-65　The buccal view of the finished preparation

Fig 5-66　The lingual view of the finished preparation

The mesial view of the finished preparation(Fig 5-67) and the distal view(Fig 5-68). The marginal line is parallel to the direction of the CEJ. The shape of the prepared surface follows the anatomical contours of the original tooth.

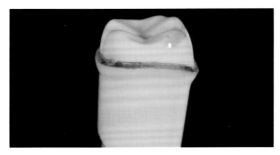 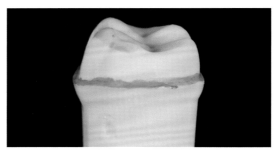

Fig 5-67　The mesial view of the finished preparation

Fig 5-68　The distal view of the finished preparation

The occlusal view of the finished preparation(Fig 5-69), which keeps the anatomical contour of the original occlusal surface.

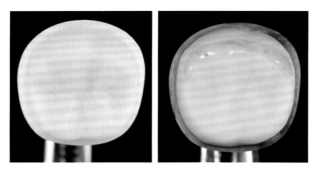

Fig 5-69　The occlusal view of the finished preparation